VAGUS & TRIGEMINAL NERVE STIMULATION

ROBERT GROYSMAN, MD

Medical Disclaimer

The information provided in this book is for educational and informational purposes only and is not intended as medical advice. The content is not a substitute for professional medical expertise or treatment. The contents of this book are not meant to diagnose, treat, or cure any illness. Always seek the advice of your physician or other qualified health providers with any questions you may have regarding a medical condition. Consult your physician if you are pregnant. Never disregard professional medical advice or delay seeking it because of something you have read in this book.

The author and publisher of this book are not responsible for any adverse effects or consequences resulting from the use of any of the suggestions, preparations, or procedures discussed in this book. All readers, especially those taking supplements, prescriptions, or over-the-counter medications, should consult their physicians before beginning any nutrition, supplement, or lifestyle program.

The information contained herein is provided "*as is*" and without warranties, either express or implied. The authors and publishers disclaim all warranties, express or implied, including, but not limited to, implied warranties of merchantability and fitness for a particular purpose. The author and publisher do not warrant or make any representations regarding the information's use, validity, accuracy, or reliability.

CONTENTS

MEDICAL DISCLAIMER 3

ABBREVIATIONS 7

MEET THE VAGUS NERVE – YOUR BODY'S "RESET BUTTON" 9
The Short Answer.. 9
What Is the Vagus Nerve? 9
What Happens When the Vagus Nerve Breaks Down? 10
How Can We Fix It? 11
The Vagus Nerve's Special Role in Inflammation 11
What's Coming Up Next? 12

MEET THE TRIGEMINAL NERVE – A SURPRISING ALLY IN RECOVERY 14
What Is the Trigeminal Nerve?... 14
Why Does It Matter in Long COVID? 15
What Is Trigeminal Nerve Stimulation (TNS)? 15
What Can TNS Help With? 16
How Does It Work? 17

NATURAL WAYS TO WAKE UP YOUR VAGUS NERVE 19
Why Stimulating the Vagus Nerve Works 20
Physical Techniques (You Can Do Anytime)....................................... 20
Lifestyle Habits That Boost Vagal Activity..................................... 21
Nutritional Tools That Support the Vagus Nerve................................. 22
Vagus Nerve Boosters 24

USING DEVICES TO STIMULATE THE VAGUS AND TRIGEMINAL NERVES 25
What Is Transcutaneous Nerve Stimulation? 25
Auricular VNS (Ear-Based).. 26
Cervical VNS (Neck-Based).. 27
Trigeminal Nerve Stimulation (TNS) Devices 29
What Stimulation Devices Are Out There? 30
How Long Does It Take to See Results?.. 32

HOW TO HANDLE SIDE EFFECTS 33
What to Expect: Normal vs. Not-So-Normal 33
Side Effects That Mean You Should Adjust Something: 34
Serious Side Effects – When to Stop and Get Help 35
How to Get Better Results (and Avoid Disappointment) 35

AVOIDING COMMON MISTAKES 36
TUNING YOUR PROTOCOL 37
WHY DO SOME PEOPLE FEEL WORSE WITH STIMULATION? **38**
HOW VAGUS AND TRIGEMINAL NERVE STIMULATION HELP YOU **43**
LONG COVID AND A NERVOUS SYSTEM OUT OF BALANCE 43
YOUR AT-HOME GUIDE TO VAGUS NERVE STIMULATION **49**
WHO SHOULD NOT USE VNS WITHOUT MEDICAL ADVICE? 53
WHAT CONDITIONS CAN TNS HELP? 56
**TRIGEMINAL NEURALGIA AND HOW EXTERNAL TRIGEMINAL NERVE
STIMULATION (TNS) CAN HELP** **63**
COMPARING EAR TO CERVICAL VAGUS NERVE STIMULATION **67**
HOW LONG CAN YOU USE A VAGUS NERVE STIMULATOR? **77**
VNS FOR MENTAL HEALTH – CALMING THE STORM WITHIN **80**
VNS FOR GUT ISSUES – HOW YOUR VAGUS NERVE CONTROLS DIGESTION **84**
VNS FOR HORMONAL BALANCE AND MENSTRUAL SYMPTOMS **89**
VNS FOR SLEEP – CALMING THE SYSTEM FOR DEEP, RESTORATIVE REST **94**
VNS VS. OTHER BRAIN & NERVE STIMULATION THERAPIES **99**
BUILDING A RECOVERY ROUTINE **104**
VNS FOR POTS – RESETTING A NERVOUS SYSTEM ON OVERDRIVE **110**
**EPIPHARYNGEAL ABRASIVE THERAPY (EAT): A GENTLE RESET FOR VAGUS AND
TRIGEMINAL NERVES** **115**
REAL PEOPLE, REAL HEALING **121**
REWIRING THE SYSTEM: HOW YOUR NERVOUS SYSTEM LEARNS TO HEAL **127**
WHAT HELPS (OR HURTS) NEUROPLASTICITY 129
ADVANCED TOOLS TO BOOST NERVE RECOVERY **132**
STUCK? HERE'S HOW TO GET UNSTUCK **138**
YOUR RECOVERY ROADMAP **143**
BUILD YOUR OWN NERVE HEALING PLAN **148**
HRV – HOW TO KNOW IF YOU'RE HEALING **154**
YOUR RECOVERY DASHBOARD **161**
STAYING BETTER FOR GOOD **166**
APPENDIX: GETTING VNS TO WORK WITHOUT THE FRUSTRATION **171**

REFERENCES **176**

Abbreviations

ALA   Alpha Lipoic Acid (a supplement)

aVNS   Auricular Vagus Nerve Stimulation (stimulation of the vagus nerve through a branch in the ear, same as taVNS)

CAIP   Cholinergic Anti-Inflammatory Pathway (an anti-inflammatory pathway in the body which is influenced by the vagus nerve)

CES   Cranial Electrotherapy Stimulation (gentle pulses to the earlobes or temples to induce a more relaxed state in the brain)

EAT   Epipharyngeal Abrasion Technique (a treatment for inflammation behind the nasal cavity that also stimulates the vagus and trigeminal nerves)

HPA   Hypothalamic-Pituitary-Adrenal Axis (part of the neuroendocrine system that controls the body's reactions to stress, which can be influenced by the vagus nerve)

HRV   Heart Rate Variability (a measure of heart rate that can be used to monitor progress of increased vagal nerve tone)

IBS	Irritable Bowel Syndrome
PBM	Photo biomodulation (the use of specific wavelengths of light to influence the cells in the body)
POTS	Postural Orthostatic Tachycardia Syndrome (a condition where the heart rate increases too much when going from lying down to standing up)
PTSD	Post-Traumatic Stress Disorder (a condition which can develop following the experience or witnessing of a traumatic event)
SIBO	Small Intestinal Bacterial Overgrowth
taVNS	Transcutaneous Auricular Vagal Nerve Stimulation (stimulation of the vagus nerve through the skin on a branch located in the ear, same as aVNS)
tcVNS	Transcutaneous Cervical Vagal Nerve Stimulation (stimulation of the vagus nerve through the skin on the neck
TNS	Trigeminal Nerve Stimulation (stimulating the trigeminal nerve)
VNS	Vagal Nerve Stimulation (stimulating the vagus nerve)

Meet the Vagus Nerve – Your Body's "Reset Button"

When you think about the parts of your body that keep you going, you probably think about your heart, lungs, or brain. But there's one unsung hero working behind the scenes that's just as important: the vagus nerve.

So what is the vagus nerve? Why is it such a big deal in Long COVID? And how can we help it help us?

The Short Answer

The vagus nerve is like your body's "rest and repair" switch. When it's working well, your heart rate slows down, your digestion runs smoothly, and your body knows how to calm itself after stress. But if this nerve isn't working right—which seems to happen in many people with Long COVID—things can go haywire. You might feel constantly wired or worn out, have digestive problems, racing heartbeats, trouble breathing, or even brain fog.

Good news: We can try to "nudge" the vagus nerve back into balance. And one of the best ways to do that is through something called **vagus nerve stimulation (VNS)**, a set of methods that encourage this nerve to do its job again.

What Is the Vagus Nerve?

The vagus nerve (pronounced VAY-gus) gets its name from the Latin word for "wandering" because it wanders all over your body. It starts at the brainstem and travels down your neck, into your chest, and all the way to your gut.

Here's what it helps control:

- **Heart rate** – slows it down when you're at rest
- **Breathing** – keeps your breathing calm and steady
- **Digestion** – helps you process food, absorb nutrients, and stay regular
- **Mood and emotions** – connects to parts of your brain that help with feeling calm and socially connected
- **Immune system** – helps reduce harmful inflammation when it's overactive

You can think of the vagus nerve as the captain of the parasympathetic nervous system, the team that helps your body calm down, heal, and recover.

What Happens When the Vagus Nerve Breaks Down?

In people with Long COVID, researchers have found that the vagus nerve can get inflamed or damaged, leading to a condition called **dysautonomia**, where the automatic systems in your body (like breathing, heart rate, digestion, and temperature control) don't work smoothly.

Some common symptoms linked to poor vagus nerve function:

- Fast or irregular heartbeat
- Feeling dizzy when standing up
- Nausea, bloating, or constipation
- Shortness of breath
- Anxiety or depression
- Fatigue that doesn't go away with rest
- Brain fog

If this sounds familiar, you're not alone. Studies show that up to **80% of people with Long COVID** have signs of vagus nerve involvement.

How Can We Fix It?

That's where **vagus nerve stimulation (VNS)** comes in.

VNS is a way to gently "tap" the vagus nerve and remind it how to do its job. It's like pressing a reset button for your body's healing system.

You can stimulate the vagus nerve in several ways:

- Breathing exercises
- Humming, singing, or chanting
- Splashing cold water on your face
- Certain kinds of acupuncture
- Special nerve stimulation devices that attach to your ear or neck

And the best part? Many of these are easy, low-cost, and can be done at home.

The Vagus Nerve's Special Role in Inflammation

One of the vagus nerve's most amazing jobs is reducing inflammation, the kind of chronic, low-level inflammation that makes you feel sick and tired.

It does this through a built-in system called the **Cholinergic Anti-Inflammatory Pathway (CAIP for short)**. When the vagus nerve is activated, it tells your immune system to tone down the release of harmful substances like TNF-α, IL-1β, and IL-6—chemicals that are often elevated in Long COVID.

In other words, a healthy vagus nerve doesn't just help you relax. It helps your entire body heal.

The vagus nerve is part of the parasympathetic nervous system. The nervous system in our body has two major settings: the "go" mode and the "rest" mode. These are controlled by two branches of what's called the **autonomic nervous system**—the part of the nervous system that runs automatically, without you needing to think about it. The **sympathetic nervous system** is responsible for the "fight or flight" response. It's what kicks in when you're stressed, scared, or in danger. It increases your heart rate, makes you breathe faster, and pumps blood to your muscles to prepare you for action.

On the other hand, the **parasympathetic nervous system** is your body's "rest and digest" mode. It helps you calm down after a stressful event, slowing your heart rate, aiding digestion, and helping the body repair itself. Think of it as the system that helps your body recover, recharge, and heal. These two systems work like a seesaw—when one is more active, the other is less so.

In a healthy body, the sympathetic and parasympathetic systems balance each other out. You need the sympathetic system to handle emergencies or meet daily challenges, but you also need the parasympathetic system to keep your body in a state of repair and long-term health. Problems arise when the "fight or flight" system stays on for too long, as it can wear down the body over time. That's why supporting your parasympathetic nervous system—through deep breathing, relaxation, sleep, or therapies like vagus nerve stimulation—can be so important for your health.

What's Coming Up Next?

In the next chapters, we'll break down:

- All the different ways you can stimulate the vagus nerve (both high-tech and natural)

- A deep dive into a similar nerve—the trigeminal nerve—and why it matters too

- How to choose the right kind of stimulation for your needs

- How to handle side effects, avoid risks, and get the most out of these treatments

- What the latest research shows about vagus nerve therapy for Long COVID

So, if you've been struggling with strange symptoms and haven't gotten answers, this might be the missing piece of the puzzle. You're not crazy. You're not imagining it. And most importantly—there is something you can do.

Meet the Trigeminal Nerve – A Surprising Ally in Recovery

You've probably heard of the vagus nerve, but there's another powerful nerve that plays a big role in how you feel—and it might be a game-changer for people with Long COVID. It's called the **trigeminal nerve**, and even though it mostly controls your face, it connects deeply with your brain and nervous system.

In fact, stimulating this nerve might help calm your body, improve sleep and mood, reduce chronic pain, and rebalance your nervous system, especially if Long COVID has thrown it out of whack.

Let's break it down in plain English.

What Is the Trigeminal Nerve?

The **trigeminal nerve** is the **fifth cranial nerve**, and it's the biggest of all the cranial nerves. Its name comes from the Latin word for "three twins," because it has three big branches:

- **Ophthalmic branch** – goes to your forehead, scalp, and upper eyelids
- **Maxillary branch** – connects to your cheeks, nose, and upper teeth
- **Mandibular branch** – runs to your jaw, lower teeth, and part of your tongue

Together, these branches control the **sensation in your face** and **muscles used for chewing**—but the trigeminal nerve does a lot more than that.

It connects to deeper brain areas involved in **pain, emotion, attention, sleep, and autonomic function** (like heart rate and digestion). That's why stimulating this nerve—called **trigeminal nerve stimulation (TNS)**—can actually help your whole body, not just your face.

Why Does It Matter in Long COVID?

In Long COVID, many people experience:

- Facial pain or numbness
- Tingling or weird sensations in the head or scalp
- TMJ (jaw tension)
- Headaches or pressure behind the eyes
- Brain fog, anxiety, insomnia

The trigeminal nerve is likely involved in a lot of these symptoms, especially when inflammation or nervous system imbalance affects the brainstem, where this nerve connects.

By gently stimulating this nerve, we can "send signals" back into the brain that may help **calm inflammation**, **reset pain pathways**, and **rebalance the autonomic nervous system** (especially the part that handles rest, digestion, and healing).

What Is Trigeminal Nerve Stimulation (TNS)?

Trigeminal Nerve Stimulation (TNS) is a non-invasive technique where small electrical pulses are applied to the skin on your **forehead**, usually above the eyebrows. These pulses target the **supraorbital** and **supratrochlear** branches of the trigeminal nerve.

It's completely **painless**, and there's no surgery or implant required. Many people use sticky pads or electrodes at home, usually for **20–30 minutes once or twice a day**.

What Can TNS Help With?

Here are some of the conditions TNS has been used for—many of which overlap with Long COVID symptoms:

Neurological

- Epilepsy (especially drug-resistant types)
- Migraine and cluster headaches

Psychiatric

- Depression (including treatment-resistant depression)
- PTSD (Post-Traumatic Stress Disorder)
- OCD

Pain

- Facial pain and TMJ
- Chronic widespread pain
- Fibromyalgia

Sleep and Cognitive Function

- Insomnia
- Poor focus or attention
- ADHD (especially in children)

Autonomic Dysfunction

- POTS (Postural Orthostatic Tachycardia Syndrome)
- Long COVID-related dysautonomia
- Unexplained fatigue or brain fog

Recovery from Brain Injury

- Stroke recovery
- Traumatic brain injury (TBI)

How Does It Work?

TNS works by gently **activating brain circuits** that control pain, mood, and nervous system balance. Here's what it may help do:

- **Calm overactive stress pathways** (sympathetic nervous system)
- **Promote healing and rest** (parasympathetic system)
- **Change how the brain responds to pain and inflammation**
- **Boost feel-good neurotransmitters** like serotonin and norepinephrine
- **Improve blood flow and brain function**

Is It Safe?

Yes—TNS is **non-invasive and well-tolerated**. Most people have no side effects, or only very mild ones like:

- Tingling at the electrode site
- Slight skin irritation
- Sleepiness (if used before bed)

Final Thoughts

The trigeminal nerve may not get as much attention as the vagus nerve, but it's just as important—especially in conditions like Long COVID. Stimulating this nerve is safe, easy, and may help reduce symptoms that medications haven't touched.

In the coming chapters, we'll dive deeper into how to use VNS and TNS at home, what to look out for, and how to adjust your approach if something isn't working.

Natural Ways to Wake Up Your Vagus Nerve

The vagus nerve is like a calming control center for your whole body. When it's working well, your heart slows down, your digestion flows smoothly, your immune system cools off, and your mind feels clear and relaxed.

Every moment, your parasympathetic and sympathetic nervous systems are scanning your environment—and your internal thoughts about it—to decide how your body should respond. This automatic process is designed to keep you safe. Ideally, your body spends most of its time in the parasympathetic state, where it can rest, digest, and heal. But trauma, chronic stress, or illnesses like viral infections can cause your nervous system to get stuck in sympathetic overdrive, where the body stays on high alert even when there's no immediate danger. This shift in baseline wiring can have powerful effects on health, mood, and recovery.

If the vagus nerve is sluggish, as it often is in **Long COVID**, those systems can go haywire.

That's the bad news.

The good news? You can help **retrain** your vagus nerve to function better and many of the tools are free, simple, and right at your fingertips.

This chapter covers **physical techniques, lifestyle habits, and nutritional tools** you can use to stimulate the vagus nerve gently and safely from home.

Why Stimulating the Vagus Nerve Works

Your vagus nerve is part of the **parasympathetic nervous system**—the part that tells your body it's safe to relax, digest, and heal. When you stimulate it, you're sending a signal to your brain that says, "We're okay. We don't need to stay in fight-or-flight mode."

This helps:

- Reduce inflammation
- Lower heart rate
- Improve digestion
- Calm the mind
- Balance hormones and immune function

Let's go through the top ways to do it.

Physical Techniques (You Can Do Anytime)

1. Deep, Slow Breathing

How: Inhale slowly for 4–6 seconds, then exhale slowly for 6–8 seconds. Do 5–10 minutes once or twice daily.

Why it works: Long, slow exhalations increase parasympathetic activity and improve heart rate variability (a marker of vagus nerve health).

Best for: Calming anxiety, lowering stress, improving focus

2. Gargling

How: Gargle warm water vigorously for 30–60 seconds.

Why it works: It stimulates throat muscles connected to the vagus nerve and activates brain pathways through the vocal cords.

Best for: Clearing brain fog, boosting tone, and waking up the nerve reflex

3. Humming, Singing, or Chanting

How: Hum for several minutes a day or sing at full volume. Chanting "OM" works well too.

Why it works: The vibrations stimulate the vagus nerve through the voice box and inner ear.

Best for: Relaxation, improving mood, and boosting vagal tone

4. Cold Water Splash or Immersion

How: Splash cold water on your face or dunk your face in a bowl of cold water for 10–20 seconds.

Why it works: This triggers the "diving reflex," which activates the vagus nerve and slows heart rate.

Best for: Sudden anxiety, panic, or to reset the nervous system

5. Valsalva Maneuver

How: Pinch your nose, close your mouth, and try to blow out like you're inflating a balloon, without letting air out. Hold for 10 seconds.

Why it works: It stimulates pressure receptors that activate the vagus nerve and helps regulate heart rate.

Best for: Brief resets of the nervous system, palpitations

Lifestyle Habits That Boost Vagal Activity

6. Meditation and Mindfulness

How: Sit quietly and focus on your breath or body sensations for 5–20 minutes.

Why it works: It reduces overactivity in stress circuits and boosts parasympathetic tone.

Best for: Stress management, improving mental clarity

7. Yoga and Tai Chi

How: Combine breath, movement, and mindfulness in a structured practice.

Why it works: These regulate the autonomic nervous system and boost vagus nerve signals.

Best for: Physical and mental balance, body awareness, recovery

8. Massage

How: Gently massage the neck, shoulders, or around the carotid artery (sides of the neck).

Why it works: This is direct stimulation of vagal nerve branches and pressure receptors.

Best for: Relaxation, tension relief, nervous system reset

9. Laughter and Positive Social Connection

How: Spend time with people who make you feel safe and laugh often. Watch a funny show if needed.

Why it works: Social engagement is part of the vagus nerve's job, especially through the "ventral vagal" system.

Best for: Emotional regulation, mood, immune health

Nutritional Tools That Support the Vagus Nerve

10. Omega-3 Fatty Acids

How: Take a fish oil supplement or eat fatty fish, like salmon, sardines, or walnuts/flaxseeds.
Why it works: It supports vagal activity and reduces inflammation through the anti-inflammatory pathway.

Best for: Long-term immune and brain health

11. Probiotics (Gut-Health Boosters)

How: Take strains like *Lactobacillus rhamnosus* or eat fermented foods like yogurt, kefir, sauerkraut.

Why it works: This supports gut-vagus communication, helping regulate mood, inflammation, and immunity.

Best for: Digestive symptoms, brain fog, mood swings

12. Intermittent Fasting

How: Eat during an 8–10 hour window each day (like 10am to 6pm) and fast the rest of the time.

Why it works: This reduces inflammation, boosts parasympathetic tone, and enhances vagal reflexes through gut rest.

Best for: Gut healing, energy reset, metabolic support

Vagus Nerve Boosters

Method	How It Helps	When to Use It
Deep Breathing	Activates parasympathetic system	Daily or during stress
Gargling / Humming	Stimulates vagus via throat/ear	Morning or pre-bed
Cold Splash / Immersion	Activates vagus via diving reflex	Acute anxiety or heart palpitations
Yoga / Meditation	Balances nervous system	Daily routine
Omega-3s / Probiotics	Support vagus via gut-immune axis	Ongoing nutrition support
Massage	Physical vagus nerve stimulation	During rest or after exercise
Intermittent Fasting	Resets vagus–gut rhythm	2–3x per week

Final Thoughts

You don't need fancy equipment or expensive therapies to begin healing your vagus nerve. These simple tools, when practiced consistently, can retrain your body's built-in healing systems—especially if Long COVID has knocked them out of rhythm.

Even small changes in your daily habits can begin to shift your nervous system from survival mode to recovery mode.

Using Devices to Stimulate the Vagus and Trigeminal Nerves

Y ou've already learned that your vagus and trigeminal nerves are key players in helping your body recover from Long COVID—calming inflammation, improving brain function, balancing your heart rate, digestion, and more.

In this chapter, we'll focus on **devices** that can help you stimulate these nerves from the outside—without surgery, needles, or implants.

We'll show you:

- What kinds of nerve stimulation devices are out there

- How to choose one (even on a budget)

- What symptoms they may help with

- How to get started safely

- What side effects to watch for and how to fix them

What Is Transcutaneous Nerve Stimulation?

"Transcutaneous" just means **through the skin**. These devices send gentle electrical pulses into the nerves—either at the **ear (auricular)** or the **neck (cervical)** for the vagus nerve, or the **forehead** for the trigeminal nerve.

You control how long and how strong the stimulation is. You usually feel a mild tingling or pulsing sensation—not pain. It's safe, adjustable, and often very effective when used regularly.

Two Main Types of Vagus Nerve Stimulation (VNS) Devices

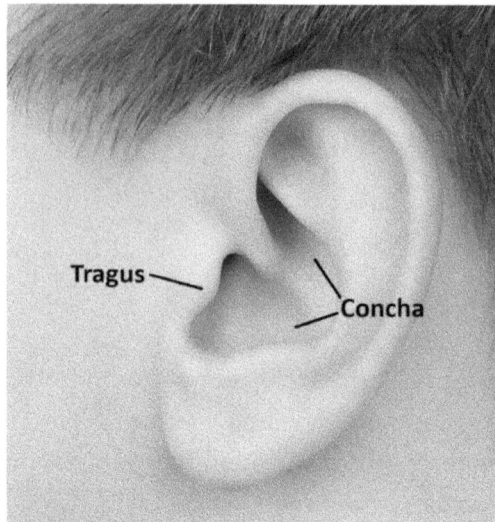

Auricular VNS (Ear-Based)

Also called taVNS or aVNS

This method uses **clips or sticky pads** on the ear, usually the tragus

or concha. These areas are connected to a small branch of the vagus nerve that runs through the ear. The tragus is also a convenient place to place a clip. You can a also cut down a a TENS skin pad to fit into the concha areas. Do not cut the wire or where the wire comes into the pad. If you use a pad you will need to change it out often since the adhesive won't last. These areas cover the vagus nerve inputs.

Pros:

- Very safe as it doesn't affect heart rate directly
- Can be worn longer (20–60 minutes)
- Easy to do at home
- Inexpensive if using a TENS unit
- Especially good for inflammation, anxiety, fatigue, and brain fog

Watch out for:

- Skin irritation (rotate placement and moisturize)
- No effect after 30 days? Try switching ear or location

Cervical VNS (Neck-Based)

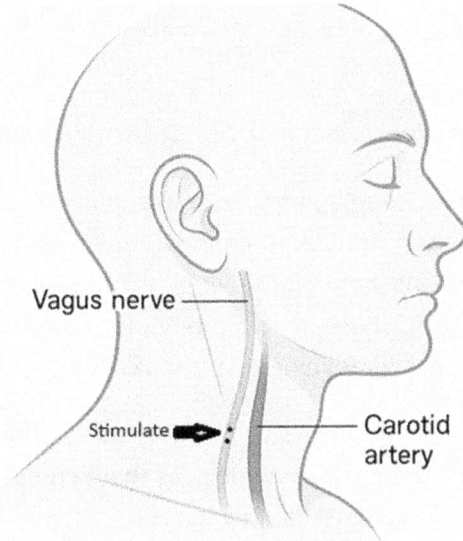

This method places the device on the **side of your neck**, over the main vagus nerve. The point of stimulation is the middle of your neck between your jaw line and your clavicle just behind the pulse of your carotid. Both pads or contact points should be applied there. To find the correct spot, feel for your carotid pulse with 1-2 fingers and put the pads just behind the carotid pulse. This stimulates **deeper pathways** that control heart rate, digestion, and more.

Pros:

- More powerful effects (when needed)
- Used for migraines, cluster headaches, and nervous system disorders
- Some people report stronger results than ear-based stimulation

Caution:

- Can lower heart rate, so this is not recommended if you have low pulse or heart issues

- Only use 1–2 times per day, for short bursts (a few minutes)

- Start slow and monitor your heart rate during use

- May cause dizziness, shortness of breath, or pressure in the chest if overused

Can Chest, Necklace, or Wrist Devices Really Stimulate the Vagus Nerve?

You might have seen ads for wearable gadgets—like vibrating necklaces, wristbands, ankle devices, or chest patches—that claim to "stimulate your vagus nerve" and help you relax, sleep better, or feel less stressed. But here's the truth: **most of these devices aren't actually stimulating the vagus nerve** in any meaningful or medical way.

Scientists have found ways to safely stimulate this nerve through the **ear** or the **side of the neck** using devices that send gentle electrical signals— this is called vagus nerve stimulation (VNS). Some of these devices are even approved by the FDA to treat things like epilepsy, depression, or migraines.

Why Wristbands, Necklaces, and Chest Devices Don't Work the Same Way

Here's the thing: **the vagus nerve doesn't run through your wrist, chest, ankle, or hand** in a way that can be reached from the outside. So if a device is vibrating in those areas, it's not directly touching or activating the vagus nerve at all.

That doesn't mean they're useless—but they **aren't doing what they claim**. The soothing vibrations might help you feel more relaxed, kind of like a gentle massage or white noise machine might. It could help with mindfulness or breathing—but that's more of a **calming or placebo effect**, not actual nerve stimulation.

What *Does* Work?

If you really want to stimulate the vagus nerve, the only proven ways to do it are:

- **Through the ear**, especially areas like the tragus or cymba conchae.
- **Through the neck**, where the vagus nerve is closer to the skin.

Devices that do this (like some approved ear clips or neck patches) have been studied in clinical trials and show real effects on the brain and body.

Examples of Devices That Don't Actually Stimulate the Vagus Nerve:

- **Apollo Neuro** (wrist): Uses vibration to promote calm, but doesn't access the vagus nerve.
- **Sensate** (chest): Vibrates on your sternum, may feel relaxing but doesn't touch the vagus nerve.
- **Other "wellness" devices** that buzz or hum on the body—these might help you feel better in the moment but aren't providing true vagus nerve stimulation.

Just because a gadget vibrates doesn't mean it's stimulating your vagus nerve. **If it's not on the ear or neck, it's not doing real vagus nerve stimulation.** It might still feel good—and that's okay! But it's important to know the difference between real nerve stimulation and just a relaxing sensation.

Trigeminal Nerve Stimulation (TNS) Devices

These devices stimulate the **forehead**, near your eyebrows. That's where two branches of the trigeminal nerve run, and sending mild pulses here can affect brain circuits that control **mood, pain, sleep, and focus**.

Used for:

- Migraines
- ADHD (FDA-cleared for children)
- PTSD, depression, and anxiety
- Brain fog and insomnia in Long COVID
- Chronic facial pain

Typical setup: Sticky pads or a headset worn on the forehead, usually 20–30 minutes once or twice per day.

What Stimulation Devices Are Out There?

Device Name	Type	Approved Use	Good For	Notes
gammaCore™	Cervical VNS	Migraines, cluster HA	Headaches, vagus tone	FDA-approved, higher cost
tVNS®	Ear VNS	Not FDA approved (EU use)	Mood, fatigue, inflammation	Easy-to-use ear clips
NEMOS®	Ear VNS	Europe: epilepsy, mood	Brain fog, Long COVID symptoms	Not sold in U.S.
TENS 7000	DIY taVNS	Not approved for vagus use	Long COVID, inflammation	Affordable, requires manual setup

Device Name	Type	Approved Use	Good For	Notes
Monarch eTNS	Trigeminal (TNS)	ADHD in kids	Brain fog, ADHD, mood	FDA-cleared, forehead placement
Neurosym Truvaga	Cervical VNS	Wellness only (not FDA)	Mood, focus, sleep	Home neck-stim device, U.S. only
Vagustim	Ear VNS	Not FDA approved	Wellbeing	Smart phone linked; unique ear piece accessory
Vagal.com	Ear VNS	Not FDA approved	Wellness	Small and phone programmable

Setting Up a DIY Auricular VNS (taVNS) with a TENS Unit

You'll need:

- A TENS unit with adjustable frequency (15–30 Hz) and pulse width (250 μs)
- Ear clip electrodes (double contact)
- Conductive gel or water
- Clean, moisturized ear (preferably the **left tragus**)
- Start with **1–3 mA** (until you feel a tingle, not pain)
- Run for **20–30 minutes once or twice a day**

Pro tips:

- Stick to the left ear for safety, the right ear connects more closely to the heart.

- Avoid the earlobe as there's no vagus nerve there.

- If the clip won't stay on, try the cymba concha instead.

- If one spot doesn't work, switch to a new area or alternate ears every few days.

- If you don't feel anything, try applying conductive gel or wetting

How Long Does It Take to See Results?

Most people begin noticing changes in **2–4 weeks**, especially with daily use. Improvements may include:

- Better sleep

- Less fatigue

- Fewer palpitations

- Reduced anxiety

- Improved brain fog

If there's no noticeable benefit after 30 days:

- Try changing the stimulation location or settings

- Use it twice a day instead of once

- Experiment with different times of day (AM vs. PM)

Final Thoughts

You don't need expensive implants to access the healing power of your vagus and trigeminal nerves. With just a bit of guidance and a simple device—or even a basic TENS unit—you can start calming your nervous system, fighting inflammation, and helping your body heal from Long COVID.

How to Handle Side Effects

Vagus nerve stimulation (VNS) and trigeminal nerve stimulation (TNS) are powerful tools. They can help reduce inflammation, regulate your heart rate and digestion, clear brain fog, and calm your body's response to stress.

But like any therapy, nerve stimulation isn't one-size-fits-all.

Some people feel amazing after the first session. Others might feel a little dizzy, too stimulated, or even worse before they feel better. That's normal—and it's often easy to fix.

This chapter will help you:

- Recognize common side effects
- Know when something is *not* normal
- Adjust your setup for better results
- Avoid common mistakes
- Troubleshoot when things don't work

What to Expect: Normal vs. Not-So-Normal

Mild Side Effects That Are Usually Okay:

These are common, especially in the first week:

Symptom	Cause	What to Do
Mild tingling or warmth	Nerve activation	No need to change anything
Slight ear redness or itchiness	Skin reaction to clip or pad	Moisturize, rotate placement
Light fatigue or sleepiness	Nervous system calming	Use stimulation before bed
Gentle drop in heart rate	Parasympathetic activation	Only use the **left ear**

Side Effects That Mean You Should Adjust Something:

These aren't dangerous, but they mean you should tweak your settings or approach:

Symptom	Likely Cause	Fix
Dizziness	Stimulation too strong	Lower intensity or shorten time
Nausea or queasiness	Overactivation of gut-brain axis	Switch to once daily or move to tragus
Sharp tingling or pain	Too much intensity or dry skin	Lower intensity, use conductive gel
Palpitations or skipped beats	Right ear or cervical overstimulation	Use **only left ear** or stop neck stimulation

Symptom	Likely Cause	Fix
Hoarseness or tight throat	Deep cervical stimulation	Lower intensity or switch to ear-only
Anxiety or wired feeling	Too frequent or late-day use	Switch to mornings only

Serious Side Effects – When to Stop and Get Help

Very rare, but important to watch for:

- Fainting or passing out
- Uncontrollable heart rate changes
- Severe breathing trouble
- Severe pain, burns, or skin damage

Stop immediately and consult a healthcare provider. These are not expected effects from properly done external vagus or trigeminal stimulation.

How to Get Better Results (and Avoid Disappointment)

Many people give up too early because they expect results overnight or don't use the device correctly. Here's how to do it right:

Use Consistently

Just like exercise, the benefits of nerve stimulation **build up over time**. Most people need:

- Daily sessions for 2–4 weeks
- 20–30 minutes per session

- For chronic conditions like Long COVID, even 2x daily use can help

Adjust If Nothing Is Happening

If you feel nothing at all after 3–4 weeks:

- Switch from the tragus to the **cymba concha**
- Try a **different ear** (but check your heart rate on the right ear!)
- Increase the **frequency** gradually (start at 20–25 Hz, then try 30 Hz)
- **Vary the time of day** (try AM and PM sessions)

Watch Your Heart Rate

If you're using **neck-based stimulation** or the **right ear**, use a smartwatch or pulse oximeter to watch for heart rate drops. If your heart rate falls below 50 or you feel faint—stop and talk to your doctor.

Avoiding Common Mistakes

Mistake	Why It's a Problem	What to Do Instead
Using earlobe instead of tragus	No vagus nerve fibers in earlobe	Use tragus or cymba concha instead
Using TENS unit on EMS/Burst mode	Wrong stimulation pattern	Set to **continuous** at 20–30 Hz
Only stimulating once a week	Not enough to retrain the nervous system	Do it daily, at least for 4 weeks
Expecting instant results	This isn't like Tylenol	Look for improvements over weeks
Not checking device specs	Not all "TENS" units allow custom settings	Use a programmable unit like TENS 7000

Only use a continuous, conventional, or normal mode. Do not use NMES units, IFC (Interferential), Functional electric stimulation (FES), or burst modes or units.

Tuning Your Protocol

Here's how to build a **simple and effective daily routine**:

Step	Details
When	Start with 1x/day, morning or before bed
Duration	20–30 minutes per session
Ear	Left ear only (tragus preferred)
Settings	25 Hz frequency, 250 µs pulse width, mild tingle
Intensity	Start at 1–3 mA (just enough to feel sensation)
Adjust after 2–4 weeks	Add second session or change placement

Summary: How to Stay Safe and Successful

- Start low and slow
- Use only the **left ear** unless supervised
- Stick with it daily as **2 to 4 weeks** is the usual response window
- Use a proper device with adjustable settings
- Don't push through pain or dizziness, instead dial it down
- Adjust placement or intensity if you're not improving

Why Do Some People Feel Worse with Stimulation?

How the Face and Jaw Nerves React During Ear-Based Vagus Nerve Stimulation (taVNS)

When you use a vagus nerve stimulation device on your ear (called **taVNS**), the goal is to gently activate a calming nerve called the **vagus nerve**. This nerve helps slow the heart rate, reduce inflammation, and support healing. The most effective places to stimulate are usually the **cymba conchae** (a hollow spot near the top of the ear canal) or the **tragus** (the small flap at the front of your ear).

But your ear is connected to more than just the vagus nerve. It's also linked to **other nerves**, especially the **trigeminal nerve**, which controls sensations in your face, jaw, and temple.

What Parts of the Ear Connect to Which Nerves?

Nerve	Area It Reaches
Vagus nerve	Cymba conchae, tragus (the main targets for taVNS)
Trigeminal nerve – jaw branch	Outer ear and temple
Trigeminal nerve – cheek branch	Lower edge of ear, cheek area
Facial nerve	Behind the ear
Neck nerves (from spine)	Earlobe and lower ear

Why Do You Sometimes Feel Facial Sensations During taVNS?

Even though you're trying to activate just the vagus nerve, the **other nerves in the ear area—especially those related to the face and jaw—can also get stimulated.**

This can happen because:

- **Vagus and facial nerves share communication centers in the brain**, so stimulating one can affect the other.
- **Electrical signals can spread**, especially if your device is turned up too high.
- Some people feel **face tingling, jaw tension, or eye twitching** during use—not because the vagus nerve is malfunctioning, but because other nerves are being accidentally triggered.

When That Might Be Helpful... or Not

Helpful (when trigeminal activation is desired):

- May improve **migraines**, **jaw pain**, or certain types of facial nerve sensitivity.

Not helpful (when it's unintentional):

- Can feel **uncomfortable** or **confusing**, especially if you're expecting only a calming effect.
- Might even cause a **stress response** if the wrong nerves are activated.

How to Make Stimulation More Comfortable

- Use **low intensity** and **short pulses** to prevent accidental stimulation.
- Try the **cymba conchae** area (upper ear) instead of the tragus if facial effects are unpleasant.
- If you **want** trigeminal nerve stimulation (e.g., for migraine relief), then you can use these effects purposefully.

Why Some People Feel Worse After taVNS

Although taVNS is supposed to help calm the nervous system, some people experience the opposite—**increased anxiety, racing thoughts, or tightness in the chest.**

This is especially common in people with:

- Long COVID
- Mast Cell Activation Syndrome (MCAS)
- PTSD or trauma history
- Sensitivities to mold, chemicals, or medications

- History of **benzodiazepine use** or imbalances in calming brain chemicals

What Might Be Happening?

Possible Cause	What Happens	Common Symptoms
Low vagus nerve tone	Body overreacts to stimulation	Agitation, insomnia
Stress centers in brain get triggered	Norepinephrine (a stress chemical) increases	Anxiety, tension
Face and jaw nerves are accidentally activated	Sensory overload	Jaw tightness, stress
Past trauma is reactivated	Brain misinterprets internal signals	Panic, emotional flashbacks
Intensity too high	System gets overwhelmed	Dizziness, pressure, chest discomfort

What You Can Do to Avoid or Reduce These Effects

- **Start slow**: Use very low settings (e.g., 0.2–0.5 mA, 1–2 Hz, 100 µs)

- **Short sessions**: Begin with just 30 seconds on each ear

- **Watch how you feel after**: If you get rebound anxiety, pause for a few days

- **Pair with calming tools**: Breathe deeply, stretch your limbs, or move gently during use

- **Stop temporarily** if you feel worse for more than 2 days

Final Thought:

If you don't feel calmer right away, it doesn't mean taVNS isn't working. Your nervous system may just be **too tense or too sensitive at the start**. Over time, as you reduce your baseline stress levels, taVNS can become more effective and comfortable.

This process is called **increasing your "window of tolerance"**—the amount of stimulation your nervous system can handle without overreacting.

How Vagus and Trigeminal Nerve Stimulation Help You

You've seen how simple tools like a TENS unit or a forehead stimulator can change the way your body feels by improving fatigue, brain fog, anxiety, heart rate, and digestion. But what's actually happening behind the scenes?

This chapter breaks down the **science of how nerve stimulation works**, in simple terms. No medical degree needed—just curiosity and an open mind.

Long COVID and a Nervous System Out of Balance

Long COVID isn't "just in your head." It's a whole-body condition that likely involves:

- **Chronic inflammation**

- **Nervous system imbalance** (called *dysautonomia*)

- **Ongoing immune overactivation**

- **Mitochondrial problems** (your energy factories stop working properly)

Your vagus and trigeminal nerves connect to the **control centers** that regulate all of those things.

That's why stimulating them—in the right way—can help your body rebalance itself.

1. The Vagus Nerve and the "Inflammation Switch"

Your vagus nerve controls something called the **Cholinergic Anti-Inflammatory Pathway**. It's your body's built-in anti-inflammatory switch.

Here's how it works:

1. **Your body detects inflammation**—like in Long COVID, where cytokines (inflammatory messengers) are often too high.

2. **Your vagus nerve sends a calming signal** to the immune system.

3. **Your immune cells respond by reducing** production of cytokines like:

   o   TNF-alpha

   o   IL-1 beta

   o   IL-6

These are some of the same cytokines elevated in **cytokine storms**, autoimmune flares, and persistent Long COVID inflammation.

When you stimulate the vagus nerve, you help **turn off the fire alarm** and let the body focus on healing.

2. The Brainstem Relay: NTS and DMV

Two brain areas are key to this calming effect:

- **Nucleus Tractus Solitarius (NTS):** the main "inbox" for the vagus nerve

- **Dorsal Motor Nucleus of the Vagus (DMV):** the "outbox" sending commands back to your body

When you stimulate your vagus or trigeminal nerve:

- You activate the NTS → which signals the DMV → which tells your organs to calm down, rest, digest, and heal.

These brainstem areas also connect to your **gut, lungs, heart, spleen**, and **limbic system** (the emotional center of your brain).

That's why nerve stimulation can improve **inflammation, digestion, breathing, heart rate**, and even **mood**.

4. Fixing Dysautonomia—the "Wiring Problem" Behind Many Symptoms

If you feel like your body is always stuck in high gear—racing heart, lightheadedness, anxiety, hot/cold swings—you may have **dysautonomia**. It means your **autonomic nervous system** is out of balance.

That's where vagus and trigeminal nerve stimulation come in.

They help by:

- **Turning down the sympathetic system** (fight-or-flight)
- **Turning up the parasympathetic system** (rest-and-digest)
- Helping your body learn how to shift between the two again (like a healthy heart rate variability)

This helps regulate:

- **Heart rate**
- **Blood pressure**
- **Breathing**
- **Digestive rhythm**
- **Sleep-wake cycles**
- **Stress tolerance**

4. Brain Benefits: Mood, Focus, and Energy

When you stimulate the **trigeminal nerve** (usually on the forehead), it connects to parts of the brain involved in:

- Emotion (amygdala, anterior cingulate cortex)

- Motivation and reward (caudate nucleus)

- Memory and cognition (hippocampus, prefrontal cortex)

- Pain processing (somatosensory cortex)

This is why trigeminal nerve stimulation (TNS) has been shown to help:

- **Depression and anxiety**

- **ADHD and brain fog**

- **Chronic pain**

- **Sleep problems**

For Long COVID patients, these symptoms are often tied together so stimulating the brain through TNS may offer relief across multiple systems.

5. Other Healing Pathways Activated by VNS/TNS

a. HPA Axis Support (Stress Hormone Regulation)

Stimulating the vagus nerve may also balance your **hypothalamic-pituitary-adrenal (HPA)** axis—the system that controls **cortisol**, your main stress hormone.

In Long COVID, this axis is often **flattened** (too little cortisol) or **overreactive** (causing crashes or wired fatigue).

VNS helps regulate cortisol, which:

- Reduces systemic inflammation

- Stabilizes energy levels

- Improves immune coordination

b. Macrophage Reset

Your immune system has two types of macrophages:

- **M1 = pro-inflammatory**
- **M2 = healing, anti-inflammatory**

VNS helps **shift macrophages from M1 to M2**, helping the body cool down and start repairing tissues.

c. Brain-Gut Communication

The vagus nerve is your **gut-brain superhighway**. Stimulating it can:

- Improve gut motility
- Reduce nausea, bloating, and IBS symptoms
- Calm overactive mast cells
- Help with post-meal fatigue or histamine flares

What About Long COVID Specifically?

Multiple studies and case series show that vagus or trigeminal nerve stimulation may help with:

Symptom	Likely Benefit from Nerve Stimulation
Fatigue	Reduced inflammation, better cell recovery
Brain fog	Improved blood flow and neurotransmitter balance
Palpitations/POTS	Autonomic rebalancing
Gut problems (bloating, reflux)	Gut-vagus regulation
Anxiety, panic, insomnia	Calmer brainstem and limbic response
Depression	Limbic circuit stimulation
Sleep problems	Parasympathetic activation

Final Thoughts

Your body has a powerful system already built in—a calming, healing, regulating pathway—and it runs right through the **vagus** and **trigeminal nerves**. In Long COVID, this system can become damaged or dysregulated.

Using non-invasive stimulation devices (like ear clips or forehead pads), we can help retrain this system and **nudge your body back into balance**.

Even better? We can often do this **at home**, safely, gently, and consistently by using the tools covered in the last chapters.

Your At-Home Guide to Vagus Nerve Stimulation

Everything you need to know to get started—safely, effectively, and affordably.

If you're ready to try vagus nerve stimulation (VNS) at home, this chapter walks you through it step by step.

You don't need to spend thousands of dollars or undergo surgery to access this powerful therapy. You can start today—right at home—using safe, simple equipment, as long as you know how to do it correctly.

Step 1: Choose Your Device

There are several types of VNS devices, but for home use, we'll focus on **transcutaneous auricular vagus nerve stimulation (taVNS)** using either:

Budget Option: TENS Unit (like TENS 7000)

- Price: Around $30–50

- Adjustable settings for frequency, pulse width, and intensity

- Requires ear clip electrodes or sticky pads

- Not FDA-approved for VNS but widely used off-label for taVNS

Mid-Range Option: Dedicated taVNS Devices

- Examples: tVNS® (Europe), Parasym, NEMOS (Europe)

- Price: $200–$600

- Designed specifically for vagus nerve stimulation

- Easy preset modes and comfortable clip systems

- May require international ordering if not available in your country

Step 2: Know Where to Stimulate

The vagus nerve has a small branch that reaches the **outer ear**, specifically:

Target Area	Notes
Tragus	Front flap of the ear near the opening; easiest to clip, well-studied
Cymba Concha	Inside curve above the ear canal; harder to access, may be more direct
Concha Cavum	Lower bowl near ear canal opening; also innervated, good backup site
Earlobe	There's no vagus nerve here so don't waste your time

Most people should start with the **left tragus** as it is safest for the heart.

Step 3: Set Your Parameters (for TENS units)

Use **only "normal" or "continuous" mode** and avoid EMS, burst, modulation, or random patterns.

Parameter	Recommended Setting
Frequency	25 Hz (range: 20–30 Hz)
Pulse width	250 microseconds (μs)
Intensity	Set just high enough to feel tingling but not painful (1–3 mA on TENS 7000). If you are sensitive, you can set just beneath where you can feel tingling.
Session length	Start with 20–30 minutes once per day. If you are sensitive, start with shorter sessions, even just a minute, until you are satisfied that you are tolerating the short sessions well, then increase very gradually.
Number of sessions	1x/day for the first week, then increase to 2x/day if tolerated

Make sure both electrodes are connected if using single contact:

For a single clip that has both contacts, it will be on the one connection point you select. If your unit is biphasic or bipolar the orientation of the single double contact clip is not important.

If you are using 2 single contact clips or if you are using a monopolar/monophasic unit then you can see which orientation works better for you. You can flip the locations of the clip or pads if the first way doesn't help or is causing side effects or problems.

If using a single ear clip, the second electrode must still go somewhere (e.g., neck, upper back, or second point on the same ear).

Troubleshooting Tips

Problem	Solution
No sensation	Wet the skin or use conductive gel
Skin redness/irritation	Rotate placement, use aloe or moisturizer
Sharp pain or burning	Lower intensity; check for dry or damaged clip
Device won't run	Make sure both leads are connected and skin contact is firm
Feeling worse after session	Lower time/intensity, and use only in morning

Sample Daily Routine (Week-by-Week)

Week	Frequency	Duration	Notes
1	1x/day	20 min	Use in morning; left tragus only
2	1–2x/day	25 min	Add evening session if tolerated
3	2x/day	30 min	Vary electrode site if needed
4+	2x/day	30 min	Evaluate: continue, change site, or taper

Tracking Your Progress

Use a simple journal or phone app to track key symptoms before and after each session:

Symptom	Track This
Fatigue	Energy 1–10 scale before/after
Brain fog	Focus/clarity 1–10 scale
Heart symptoms	Track heart rate (with smartwatch/pulse ox)
Gut symptoms	Bloating, motility, nausea changes
Mood/Anxiety	Calmness 1–10; panic episodes per week
Sleep	Time to fall asleep, number of wake-ups

Review your log every 1–2 weeks to see trends—small, gradual improvements matter!

Who Should NOT Use VNS Without Medical Advice?

- People with **pacemakers or defibrillators**

- People with **serious heart rhythm issues** - If your heartbeat is too fast, too slow, or irregular in a way that affects your health (like atrial fibrillation or heart block), VNS could interfere with your heart's electrical signals and make things worse. Always talk to your doctor first before starting stimulation to ensure it is safe to do so.

- Pregnant women (limited data)

- People prone to **seizures**, unless supervised

- Children, unless under medical care

If unsure, talk to your doctor before starting.

Bonus: How to Keep Progress Going

✓ Keep consistent: It's not magic, it's **training** your nervous system
✓ Tweak your setup every few weeks to prevent adaptation
✓ Pair with breathing, mindfulness, or gentle movement for better results
✓ Celebrate small wins: less brain fog, fewer crashes, calmer days
✓ Combine with other therapies as guided (diet, pacing, EAT, supplements)

Trigeminal Nerve Stimulation is a Powerful Tool for Brain and Body Healing

So far, we've focused on the **vagus nerve**, the master switch for calming your body and reducing inflammation. But it's not the only nerve that can help reset your nervous system.

Another major pathway is the **trigeminal nerve**, and it's just as important—especially for people dealing with **Long COVID symptoms** like:

- Brain fog
- Sleep problems
- Migraines or facial pain
- Mood swings or anxiety
- Poor focus or ADHD-like symptoms

In this chapter, you'll learn:

- What the trigeminal nerve does
- How stimulating it can help heal your brain
- Who should consider trigeminal nerve stimulation (TNS)
- How to do it at home safely and effectively

What Is the Trigeminal Nerve?

The **trigeminal nerve** is the 5th cranial nerve, and it's the largest. It branches across your face, forehead, nose, and jaw. It carries signals between your brain and your:

- Skin (touch, pain, pressure)
- Muscles (chewing, facial movement)
- Brain centers that process pain, emotion, and attention

When you stimulate this nerve gently, it sends a signal up into the brain—especially into areas that control **mood, energy, memory, pain, and sleep**.

How Does Trigeminal Nerve Stimulation (TNS) Work?

TNS sends gentle electrical pulses into the **forehead area**, where branches of the trigeminal nerve run just under the skin. These pulses:

- Activate brain regions like the **prefrontal cortex**, **amygdala**, and **anterior cingulate cortex**
- Modulate pain signals
- Improve emotional stability
- Enhance attention, focus, and memory
- Boost parasympathetic activity (rest-and-digest mode)

In Long COVID, where the nervous system is often dysregulated, TNS may help **restore balance** and **reduce neuroinflammation**.

What Conditions Can TNS Help?

TNS has been studied in—and often approved for—the following conditions:

Condition	Why TNS Helps
ADHD (especially in kids)	Boosts prefrontal activity and focus
Depression and anxiety	Regulates mood circuits and stress reactivity
Sleep problems / insomnia	Activates calming brain areas
Migraines and facial pain	Reduces pain signals through brainstem modulation
Post-COVID brain fog & fatigue	Improves alertness, memory, and emotional regulation
PTSD / trauma	Calms overactive threat centers (like the amygdala)
Fibromyalgia or chronic pain	Modulates pain perception and tension
Trigeminal neuralgia	Damps overactive trigeminal nerve firing and brainstem pain transmission, reducing sharp or trigger-evoked facial pain

How to Do TNS at Home

Trigeminal nerve stimulation is non-invasive and can be done with simple equipment—no surgery, no implants.

Device Options

Device	Description	Cost Range
Monarch eTNS System	FDA-cleared for kids with ADHD (ages 7–12)	~$900+
Generic TENS units like TENS 7000	Use sticky pads on the forehead; set correct parameters	~$30–$60
CES devices (e.g. Alpha-Stim)	Similar effect; clips on earlobes, works systemically	~$500–$1,000

Where to Place the Electrodes

You want to stimulate the **supraorbital and supratrochlear branches** of the trigeminal nerve:

- Place **two sticky electrodes** just above your eyebrows, about an inch apart.

- Or, use a **headband-style** electrode pad that wraps across your forehead.

  If both sides of your face are affected, use this placement for supraorbital:

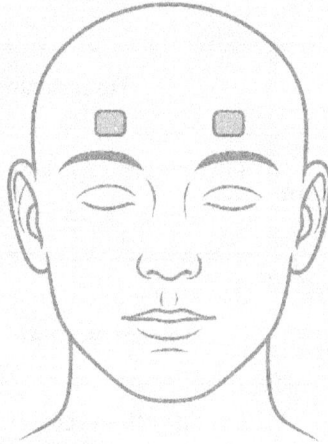

If only one side of your face is affected, place both pads on one side like this:

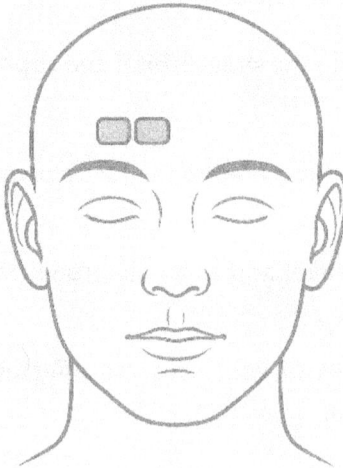

Avoid placing pads:

- Too close to your eyes or across one eye (one pad on either side of the same eye).

- On the temples

- On open or irritated skin

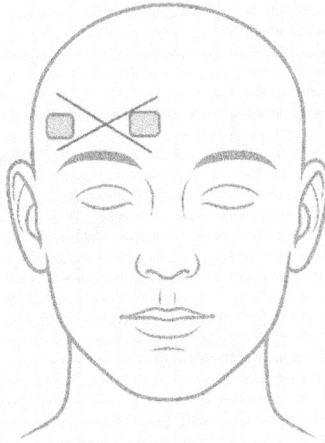

For Trigeminal nerve stimulation (TNS)

Recommended TNS Settings (Using a TENS Unit)

Parameter	Recommended Setting
Frequency	120 Hz (for pain/sleep); 1–10 Hz (for focus/mood)
Pulse width	200–250 microseconds
Intensity	Light tingling sensation or just slightly lower for very sensitive people. Keep it low enough so there is no pain.
Duration	20–30 minutes, less for very sensitive people, even for a minute or two, which can be ramped up as well-tolerated
Frequency	Once or twice daily, ideally morning and/or before bed

Most people feel relaxed after a session while others feel sharper and more focused. Track how you feel and adjust timing accordingly.

Safety Tips

TNS is considered **very safe** when done properly.

Risk	How to Avoid It
Skin irritation	Rotate pad position; clean skin before use
Dizziness or headache	Lower intensity or shorten session
Eye twitching or discomfort	Pads may be too close to eyes—reposition
Overuse fatigue	Stick to 1–2x per day unless guided otherwise

Do not use if you:

- Have a **pacemaker** or other implanted electrical device
- Are **pregnant** (without doctor approval)
- Have **epilepsy** (unless under medical supervision)

You can also stimulate the mandibular zone and the maxillary zone if you like. The maxillary zone is stimulated on the cheek with both pads on one side and the mandibular zone can be stimulated wit the pads over the jaw both pads on one side. All of these will stimulate the main trigeminal nerve.

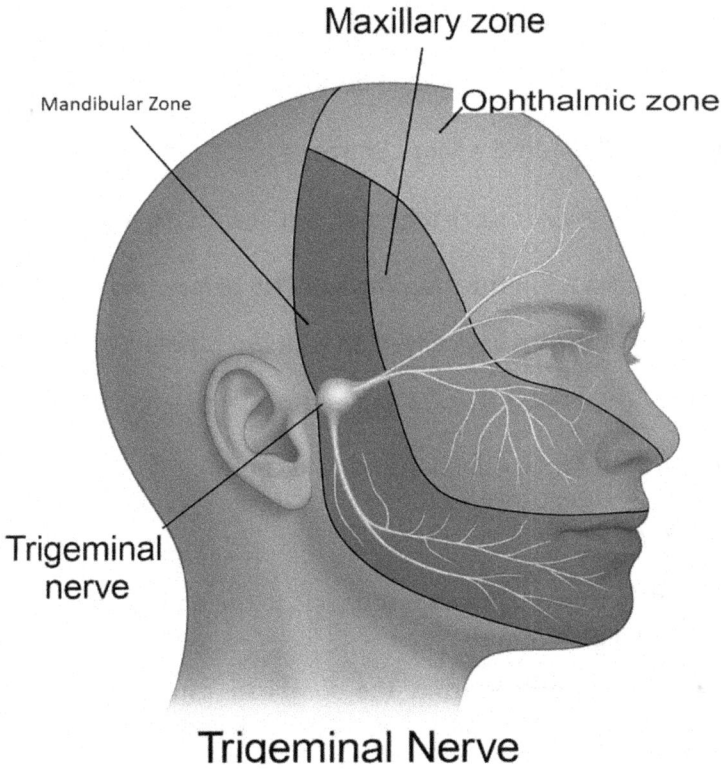

Maxillary zone

Ophthalmic zone

Mandibular Zone

Trigeminal
nerve

Trigeminal Nerve

What to Expect Over Time

Like vagus nerve stimulation, the benefits of TNS build over time.

Timeline	What You Might Notice
First week	Better sleep, calmer mood, slight brain boost
2–3 weeks	Less brain fog, more consistent energy
4+ weeks	Clearer thinking, more focus, fewer crashes

If you don't notice improvement after 3–4 weeks:

- Try using it twice daily

- Adjust frequency (e.g., 1 Hz vs. 120 Hz)

- Try a different forehead position

Combining TNS + VNS = More Power

These two therapies work **together**, not against each other. You can:

- Do **taVNS in the morning** and **TNS before bed**

- Or alternate days based on your symptoms

✓ VNS = better inflammation and autonomic function

✓ TNS = better brain function and pain control

Summary

- The **trigeminal nerve** connects to the brain's emotional, cognitive, and pain centers.

- **Stimulating it from the forehead** can help with Long COVID symptoms like brain fog, fatigue, migraines, and mood swings.

- It's safe, non-invasive, and easy to do at home using a TENS unit or a dedicated device.

- Start slow, track your results, and be consistent—your nervous system can learn and heal.

Trigeminal Neuralgia and How External Trigeminal Nerve Stimulation (TNS) Can Help

I f you've ever felt sharp, electric-like pain on one side of your face triggered by something as simple as brushing your teeth, talking, or feeling a cool breeze, you may already know the agony of **Trigeminal Neuralgia (TN)**. This condition happens when the **trigeminal nerve**, the main sensory nerve of the face, becomes **irritable or over-reactive**, sending pain signals to the brain even when there's no real danger.

Many people describe the pain as sudden lightning bolts that come and go in seconds but can repeat dozens of times a day. Traditional medications like carbamazepine can help, but they may not work for everyone or can cause side effects like dizziness, fatigue, or fogginess. That's where **external trigeminal nerve stimulation (TNS)**, a gentle, drug-free approach, can make a difference.

What Is External Trigeminal Nerve Stimulation?

External TNS is a non-invasive way to calm the overactive pain circuits in the trigeminal nerve. It uses **small adhesive pads (electrodes)** placed on the skin over the painful area, usually the **cheek (V2)** or **jawline (V3)**, connected to a small handheld device that sends gentle electrical pulses.

You'll feel a light tingling or buzzing sensation, not pain. These signals travel through the skin and influence the nerve beneath it, helping "reset" its activity and reduce the intensity of pain messages reaching the brainstem.

Think of it as **soothing static on a radio**. The electrical stimulation can "jam" excessive nerve firing and retrain the brain's pain centers to quiet down over time.

How Does It Work?

External TNS helps in several ways:

1. **Interrupting Pain Signals:**
   The mild electrical pulses interfere with the transmission of pain impulses along the trigeminal nerve, reducing the number of "pain alarms" reaching your brain.

2. **Calming Brainstem Pain Centers:**
   The trigeminal nerve connects to areas in the brainstem that process facial pain. Regular stimulation helps reduce overactivity in these circuits.

3. **Boosting Natural Pain Control:**
   TNS activates your body's own pain-relief systems, encouraging the release of endorphins and other calming neurotransmitters.

4. **Improving Nerve Balance Over Time:**
   With repeated sessions, the nerve becomes less excitable and more stable, helping prevent future flare-ups.

What to Expect During a Session

A typical TNS session lasts about **30 to 45 minutes**, done once or twice a day. You can do it at home using a portable TENS or TNS unit.

Here's what it looks like:

- Place one electrode pad over the area where the pain is felt, such as on your cheek if the pain is in the upper jaw area.

- Place the second pad a little higher up toward the temple or jawline to complete the circuit.

- Turn on the device and slowly increase the intensity until you feel a steady, comfortable tingling.

- Sit quietly, relax your face, and breathe slowly. Most people find it soothing once they get used to the sensation.

It should **never feel painful or make muscles twitch strongly**. If it does, turn the intensity down or reposition the pads.

How Often Should You Use It?

Start with:

- **1–2 sessions per day**, each lasting 30–45 minutes
- **At least 2 weeks** of consistent use before judging results

Some people notice improvement within a few days, while others need a few weeks for the nerve to settle.

What Results to Expect

- Fewer or less intense pain attacks
- Reduced need for pain medication
- Longer pain-free intervals
- Better sleep and less anxiety about flare-ups

For most people, the relief builds gradually. TNS doesn't numb the face— it helps **retrain the nerve** so it stops overreacting to normal sensations.

Safety Tips

External TNS is considered **very safe** when used correctly:

- Avoid placing pads over **open wounds, broken skin, or near the eyes**.
- Don't use it if you have a **pacemaker or implanted electrical device** unless cleared by your doctor.
- If you feel dizzy, light-headed, or your heart rate slows noticeably, stop the session and tell your provider. This is rare but possible because the trigeminal nerve connects with the vagus nerve, which influences heart rhythm.

When to Seek Professional Help

If you still have frequent, severe shocks after several weeks of regular use, talk to your doctor. Sometimes adjusting pad positions or trying a different nerve branch (V1 vs V2 vs V3) can help.
In more resistant cases, a **temporary implanted nerve stimulator** may be considered by a pain specialist, but most people start with external TNS because it's simple, safe, and inexpensive.

Key Takeaway

External trigeminal nerve stimulation gives people with Trigeminal Neuralgia a **non-drug, non-surgical tool** to calm the face's pain pathways. It works by teaching the nerve and brain to stop overreacting to normal touch or temperature, restoring calm where there once was chaos.
Used regularly and correctly, it can become a cornerstone of your daily self-care plan—helping you reclaim comfort, confidence, and peace of mind.

Comparing Ear to Cervical Vagus Nerve Stimulation

Vagus nerve stimulation (VNS) is gaining attention as a non-invasive therapy for conditions like anxiety, depression, dysautonomia, and Long COVID. Two major non-implanted VNS methods have emerged:

- **Transauricular VNS (taVNS)** – stimulation at the **ear**
- **Transcervical VNS (tcVNS)** – stimulation at the **side of the neck**

Both target parasympathetic activation but differ in their depth of nerve access, practicality, and biological effects.

What Is taVNS?

taVNS stimulates the **auricular branch** of the vagus nerve via electrodes on the **outer ear** (commonly tragus or cymba conchae).

- **Devices**: Look like earbuds or ear clips.
- **Mechanism**: Afferent signals project to the **nucleus tractus solitarius (NTS)**, a key brainstem hub.
- **Use**: 15–60 minutes per day, ideal for at-home daily neuromodulation.

Applications in Long COVID:

- Promotes **autonomic balance** (especially in POTS).

- Modulates **limbic circuits**, helping with **anxiety, depression, brain fog**.

- Safe for long-term use in **fatigue syndromes**.

- More effective for **central symptoms** (sleep, mood, cognition) than for systemic inflammation.

What Is tcVNS?

tcVNS targets the **cervical vagus nerve** through the skin of the **neck**, typically over the carotid sheath.

- **Devices**: Handheld (e.g., gammaCore®), activated in 2–3 minute bursts.

- **Mechanism**: Stimulates both afferent and **efferent vagal fibers**, affecting heart rate, inflammation, and pain.

- **Use**: 2–6 stimulations/day, especially useful for acute symptoms.

Applications in Long COVID:

- Stronger **anti-inflammatory effects** via the **cholinergic anti-inflammatory pathway**.

- More effective for **headaches, immune flares**, and elevated **IL-6 or CRP**.

- Helps manage **migraines, autoimmune features**, and cytokine-related fatigue.

- Risk of **bradycardia** and **hoarseness** in sensitive individuals.

The taVNS on the ear is more useful for long covid because:

Head-to-Head Comparison

Feature	taVNS (Ear)	tcVNS (Neck)
Access Point	Auricular branch (skin-level)	Cervical vagus (deep tissue)
Device Style	Ear clips / earbuds	Handheld device with gel
Ease of Use	Wearable during tasks	Requires active use and placement
Targeted Brain Regions	NTS, limbic, prefrontal	NTS, brainstem autonomic nuclei
Anti-inflammatory Action	Central modulation (modest)	Direct systemic immune signaling
Heart Rate Modulation	Mild	Stronger (bradycardia possible)
Treatment Time	15–60 min/day	2–3 min bursts, 2–6x/day
Approved Indications	Experimental	gammaCore®: migraines, cluster headaches
Cost	Low / DIY options	High (often $600+)

Feature	taVNS (Ear)	tcVNS (Neck)
Comfort & Tolerability	High	May cause local discomfort or hoarseness

Advantages of Each

taVNS (ear)

- **Affordable** and widely available
- Great for **daily pacing**, HRV improvement, and fatigue
- Helps with **insomnia, anxiety, brain fog**
- Suitable for **DIY or home protocols**

tcVNS (neck)

- **Deeper access** to vagus fibers
- Useful for **inflammation, migraines**, and **immune dysregulation**
- Rapid relief during **autonomic or immune flares**
- Validated in pain and inflammatory syndromes

Disadvantages of Each

taVNS (ear)

- May not reach **systemic vagal reflexes** (e.g., spleen, gut)
- Inconsistent device quality
- Slower symptom modulation in severe cases

tcVNS (neck)

- Higher cost and less accessible
- Requires **precise technique**
- Not designed for continuous stimulation
- Potential side effects in **vagal-sensitive** individuals

Side Effects Overview

Symptom	taVNS (ear)	tcVNS (neck)
Skin irritation	Occasional	Rare
Dizziness	Rare	Sometimes
Tingling	Mild (ear)	Mild to moderate (neck)
Hoarseness	Very rare	More common
Bradycardia	Rare	More likely
Headache	Rare	Rare

Caution: Avoid in patients with pacemakers, arrhythmias, or seizure disorders unless medically supervised.

Clinical Use in Long COVID

Scenario	Best Choice
Daily neuromodulation for **fatigue, anxiety, POTS, brain fog**	**taVNS**
Targeted control of **inflammation, IL-6, TNF, or migraines**	**tcVNS**
Home-based, low-cost regimen	**taVNS**
Rapid, on-demand symptom relief (flares)	**tcVNS**

taVNS vs. tcVNS

Category	taVNS (Ear Stimulation)	tcVNS (Neck Stimulation)
Advantages	- Affordable & accessible	- Deeper vagus nerve access
	- Safe for daily use	- Clinically approved for migraines & cluster headaches
	- Flexible usage (can wear during activities)	- Better access to anti-inflammatory pathways (e.g., spleen axis)
	- Ideal for long-term neuromodulation (fatigue, anxiety, brain fog)	- Helpful for acute symptom spikes or inflammatory flares

Category	taVNS (Ear Stimulation)	tcVNS (Neck Stimulation)
Disadvantages	- Targets only a small superficial branch of the vagus nerve	- Higher cost
	- Effects may be subtle in severe cases	- Requires precise neck placement with conductive gel
	- Device quality and effectiveness may vary	- Possible hoarseness, dizziness, or bradycardia
		- Not designed for continuous, all-day use

Why taVNS Is Often More Useful for Long COVID

1. Extended Daily Stimulation Promotes Repair and Regulation

- taVNS can be safely used for **30 minutes to an hour daily or even multiple times per day.**

- This **chronic stimulation** helps **retrain the autonomic nervous system**, increasing **parasympathetic tone** over time—a key deficit in Long COVID.

- Sustained stimulation is ideal for promoting **healing, neuroplasticity, and homeostatic repair** of systems dysregulated by viral injury and persistent inflammation.

2. Targets Central Nervous System Dysregulation

- The auricular branch of the vagus nerve projects to the **nucleus tractus solitarius (NTS),** which has extensive connections to:

- o The **hypothalamus** (hormone regulation)

- o **Amygdala** and **insula** (anxiety, fear, and pain perception)

- o **Prefrontal cortex** (cognition and executive function)

- This makes taVNS particularly effective for addressing **neuroinflammation, brain fog, anxiety, dysregulated sleep**, and **fatigue**, which are hallmark Long COVID symptoms.

3. Safe for All-Day Use and Gradual Titration

- Unlike tcVNS, which is designed for **short bursts** and can carry **cardiovascular risks** (e.g., bradycardia), taVNS can be used for **longer sessions with minimal risk**.

- This makes it suitable for **slow titration and neuromodulation**, which is critical in sensitive patients with:

  - o **Post-exertional malaise (PEM)**

  - o **MCAS/histamine issues**

  - o **Hypersensitivity to overstimulation**

4. Better for Fatigue, Brain Fog, and Pacing

- taVNS is more helpful in **energy conservation** and **autonomic pacing**, allowing people to use it **while resting, working, or meditating**.

- Helps with **chronic fatigue, postural orthostatic tachycardia syndrome (POTS)**, and **mental clarity**, without requiring effort or upright posture like tcVNS might.

5. More Affordable and Accessible

- taVNS devices are **widely available**, often **$100 or less**, and can be integrated into DIY or clinical protocols.

- tcVNS devices (e.g., gammaCore®) are often **cost-prohibitive**, require **prescriptions**, and are **not covered by insurance** for Long COVID.

6. Lower Risk of Side Effects

- taVNS does **not directly stimulate motor vagus fibers** that affect the **larynx and heart**, making it less likely to cause:
    - **Hoarseness**
    - **Throat tightness**
    - **Bradycardia or hypotension**
- This is especially important for **dysautonomia patients**, where **overactivation** of vagal efferents can worsen symptoms.

7. Supports Gentle Rebalancing Instead of Shock Modulation

- Long COVID is a **chronic, multisystem syndrome** that benefits more from **gentle parasympathetic nudging** than from **brief bursts of stimulation**.
- taVNS offers this **gradual neuromodulation** instead of the more intense but short-lived effects of tcVNS.

Why taVNS Is Better Suited for Long COVID?

Advantage	taVNS	Why It Matters for Long COVID
Duration	30–60+ minutes/day	Sustained parasympathetic tone promotes healing
Safety	High	Well-tolerated even in sensitive dysautonomia patients
CNS Targeting	Strong NTS, limbic, cognitive modulation	Supports mood, sleep, brain fog, fatigue
Affordability	Low cost, easy access	Suitable for long-term use and self-care
Flexibility	Can use during rest or daily activities	Helps with pacing and energy management
Side Effects	Minimal	No significant cardiac or laryngeal risks

Final Thoughts

taVNS and tcVNS are **complementary tools**, not competitors. In Long COVID, starting with **taVNS** provides a safe, accessible foundation for parasympathetic recovery. For patients with **inflammatory symptoms**, **tcVNS** may offer deeper, faster immune modulation.

In many cases, a **combined protocol**—daily taVNS plus situational tcVNS—delivers the most robust outcomes.

How Long Can You Use a Vagus Nerve Stimulator?

If you're using a vagus nerve stimulator (VNS)—whether it clips to your ear, rests on your neck, or sits behind your ear—you might be wondering: **How long is it safe to keep using it?**

The short answer is:

You can usually use it every day, for weeks, months, or even years—safely.

Let's break it down.

Is There a Time Limit?

Unlike some medications that lose effectiveness or come with long-term risks, **non-invasive vagus nerve stimulation is often safe to use long-term**. Some people use these devices daily for anxiety, depression, migraines, or Long COVID—and find that the longer they use them, the better they feel.

Think of it like physical therapy or meditation:

The more consistently you do it, the more your nervous system "learns" how to stay calm and balanced.

How Often Should You Use It?

Most people benefit from **1–2 sessions per day**.

A typical session lasts **15 to 60 minutes**, depending on your device and what you're treating.

Here are some examples:

Condition	Frequency	Typical Session Length
Anxiety or Stress	Daily or 2x daily	15–30 minutes
Long COVID	Daily	30–60 minutes
Migraines	At first sign of symptoms or daily for prevention	15–30 minutes
Poor Sleep	1 hour before bedtime	20–40 minutes

You don't need to wear the device all day. Just like going to the gym, a little regular use can go a long way.

Can You Use It Too Much?

Yes—**more is not always better**.

Using a vagus nerve stimulator too often or with settings that are too strong can lead to side effects like:

- Feeling lightheaded or dizzy

- A drop in heart rate or blood pressure

- Fatigue or feeling overly relaxed

- Tingling or irritation at the site of stimulation

If this happens, **lower the intensity** or **shorten your sessions**. Some people find that even short, gentle sessions are enough.

Do You Ever Need to Take a Break?

You might choose to take breaks if:

- Your symptoms improve and stay better for weeks
- You're trying to see if your body can maintain balance without it
- You want to check if it's really making a difference

There's no rule saying you must take breaks, but it's okay to **pause and see how you feel**. Just like you might stop a vitamin or medication to reassess, you can do the same with VNS.

Are There People Who Should Be Cautious?

Yes—some people should check with their doctor before using a VNS device:

- If you have a **very low resting heart rate**
- If you have **a pacemaker or implanted defibrillator**
- If you take medications that slow the heart (like beta-blockers)

Long-Term Use Is Safe and Common

In summary:

- Most people can use VNS daily for as long as they want
- Many feel better with consistent use over weeks and months
- It's gentle, non-invasive, and generally safe for long-term use

If you're finding benefit, there's no reason to stop—just keep listening to your body, go slowly with increases, and adjust as needed.

VNS for Mental Health – Calming the Storm Within

How vagus nerve stimulation can ease anxiety, lift mood, and quiet trauma

The Emotional Nervous System

If you've ever felt your heart race when anxious, your gut twist when stressed, or your mind shut down under pressure—that's your **autonomic nervous system** reacting to emotional triggers. And at the center of that system is the **vagus nerve**.

What many don't realize is that **mental health isn't just about brain chemistry—it's also about nerve signaling**. And VNS can directly target the circuits that shape mood, fear, and emotional resilience.

The Emotional Pathways VNS Reaches

VNS connects to brain regions that **regulate emotion, attention, and fear**, including:

- **Amygdala** – the fear and threat center
- **Hippocampus** – memory and emotional learning
- **Prefrontal cortex** – executive control and mood regulation
- **Anterior cingulate cortex** – pain, empathy, and stress response

Stimulating the vagus nerve can help **normalize activity** in these regions by reducing overreaction, calming anxiety, and improving emotional stability.

Evidence: What the Research Shows

Condition	Study Findings
Depression	VNS (especially left-sided taVNS) improves treatment-resistant depression, even in patients who failed multiple medications.
Anxiety	Studies show taVNS reduces heart rate and improves parasympathetic tone, lowering anxiety symptoms.
PTSD	VNS helps reduce hyperarousal and reactivity; improves sleep and emotional regulation.
Long COVID	Many patients experience trauma-like symptoms or post-viral mood changes; VNS supports nervous system reset.

Notably, **taVNS is now being studied as an alternative to antidepressants** in some clinical trials due to its effect on vagal tone and brain circuitry.

How VNS Calms Anxiety and Panic

When the body is **stuck in sympathetic overdrive**, your brain reads this as danger—even when there is none.

VNS helps shift the balance toward **parasympathetic dominance**, which:

- Slows heart rate
- Reduces cortisol and norepinephrine
- Improves emotional flexibility
- Enhances feelings of safety (ventral vagal activation)

This is especially helpful for people with **panic attacks, social anxiety, or trauma triggers**.

How It Compares to Medications

Feature	Medications	taVNS
Time to effect	2–6 weeks	Days to weeks
Side effects	GI issues, sedation, weight gain	Mild tingling, occasional headache
Mechanism	Neurotransmitter manipulation	Direct autonomic and brainstem modulation
Withdrawal issues	Yes (many SSRIs, benzodiazepines)	No known withdrawal
FDA approval for depression	Yes (implanted VNS)	Research and clinical use growing

Sample Protocol for Mood and Anxiety

Parameter	Recommendation
Side	Left ear (tragus or cymba concha)
Frequency	25 Hz
Pulse width	250 μs
Session time	15–30 minutes, once or twice per day
Duration	At least 4 weeks to evaluate effect
Optional add-ons	Breathwork, meditation after session

Signs of Positive Response

- Less internal tension or racing thoughts

- Reduced startle reflex or emotional reactivity

- Improved sleep and focus

- Fewer dips into panic or hopelessness

- Easier access to calm states (ventral vagal)

When to Be Cautious

- **If you feel worse** (more anxiety, dizziness, sleep disturbance): reduce intensity or shorten sessions

- **Avoid right ear stimulation** in anxious patients with low resting heart rate

- Use as a **tool**, not a crutch—combine with therapy, movement, and connection

Summary

Vagus nerve stimulation gives you access to the **body's built-in emotional regulation system**—without medication.

By calming overactive circuits and restoring balance, VNS may help treat:

- Anxiety

- Depression

- Trauma

- Emotional instability from Long COVID or dysautonomia

You're not just managing symptoms; you're retraining your nervous system to feel safe again.

VNS for Gut Issues – How Your Vagus Nerve Controls Digestion

Using vagus nerve stimulation to ease IBS, nausea, bloating, and gut inflammation

If your belly is constantly in knots, your digestion feels unpredictable, or you battle bloating, gas, and nausea after nearly every meal—you're not alone.

Digestive issues are **some of the most common symptoms** in Long COVID, dysautonomia, and POTS. And one of the biggest reasons is **vagus nerve dysfunction**.

But here's the good news: by stimulating the vagus nerve, you may be able to **reset the gut-brain connection** and help digestion run smoothly again.

How the Vagus Nerve Controls the Gut

The vagus nerve is the **main communication highway** between your brain and your gut. About **80% of the signals go from gut to brain**, and the rest go the other way.

Vagus functions in the gut:

- Increases **stomach acid and digestive enzyme release**
- Activates **gut motility** (peristalsis, the movement of food)
- Coordinates signals from the **gut microbiome** to the brain
- Detects inflammation and triggers repair

When vagal tone is low—due to viral injury, inflammation, or stress—digestion slows down, and **food just sits** in the GI tract.

Symptoms of Vagus Nerve Dysfunction in the Gut

Symptom	Why It Happens
Bloating / gas	Poor motility = fermentation / buildup
Nausea	Delayed gastric emptying / vagal shutdown
IBS symptoms (diarrhea/constipation)	Loss of gut-brain rhythm
Acid reflux or fullness	Impaired sphincter tone + slow digestion
SIBO	Poor motility allows bacterial overgrowth
Food intolerance	Sensitized gut lining, poor digestion

In many cases, the gut symptoms aren't caused by food, they're caused by **nerve miscommunication**.

How VNS Can Help Restore the Gut-Brain Loop

Stimulating the vagus nerve may:

- Increase **stomach acid and enzyme secretion**
- Reactivate **normal motility** (MMC – migrating motor complex)
- Reduce **visceral hypersensitivity** (pain from normal digestion)

- Lower gut **inflammation** via the **cholinergic anti-inflammatory pathway (CAIP)**
- Recalibrate the gut-brain axis to handle food signals calmly

Several studies have shown improvements in **gastroparesis, IBS, and gut pain** with vagus stimulation.

Evidence Snapshot

Condition	VNS Impact
IBS	Reduces gut pain, normalizes bowel movements
Gastroparesis	Improves gastric emptying and reduces nausea
SIBO	Enhances motility to prevent bacterial buildup
Gut Inflammation	Dampens TNF-alpha, IL-6 via vagal anti-inflammatory reflex

Studies also show improved **microbiome balance** after vagal stimulation which is likely due to better motility and mucosal immunity.

Protocol Tips for Digestive Recovery

Parameter	Digestive-Friendly Settings
Timing	30–60 minutes before meals (if tolerated)
Frequency	25 Hz
Pulse Width	250 µs
Side	Start with **left ear** to avoid heart effects

Parameter	Digestive-Friendly Settings
Session time	15–30 minutes
Position	Seated or reclined, not fully lying down

Be consistent. The gut loves rhythm, and daily sessions help re-establish healthy patterns.

Combine VNS With Other Gut-Calming Strategies

Tool	Why It Helps
Prokinetics (e.g., ginger, low-dose erythromycin)	Support gut movement
Butyrate/prebiotics	Rebuild gut lining and microbial balance
Herbs that calm the nervous system such as (lemon balm, chamomile)	Calm gut nerves
Deep breathing/meditation	Enhances vagal tone and gut-brain signaling
Low histamine/anti-inflammatory diet	Reduces overload on gut lining

Think of VNS as the **electrical reboot**, and these tools as the **software support**.

What If VNS Makes Gut Symptoms Worse?

Some sensitive patients report:

- Slight nausea during stimulation
- Temporary gut gurgling or cramping
- Slower bowel movements early on

These usually pass as your system **readjusts to new signals**. Try:

- Lowering intensity or session time
- Switching to **midday** or **non-meal timing**
- Using calming breathwork first to ease into stimulation

Summary

Your digestion depends heavily on **good vagal tone**. Without it, even the best diet may not digest properly.

By restoring communication between the brain and gut, **VNS may improve**:

- Nausea
- IBS
- Bloating
- SIBO
- Post-meal fatigue
- Food sensitivities

You may not have a broken gut—you may have a misfiring nerve.

And that's something you can help reset.

VNS for Hormonal Balance and Menstrual Symptoms

How vagus nerve stimulation may help regulate periods, ease PMS, and support hormone recovery

You might be surprised to learn that your **nervous system and hormones are deeply connected**—especially through the **vagus nerve**.

If you've noticed your symptoms get worse around your period...

If your cycles became irregular after COVID...

If you feel more anxious, bloated, or fatigued in the second half of your cycle...
You're not imagining it.

These changes are often signs of **dysautonomia impacting hormone balance**. The vagus nerve helps regulate many of the systems that affect estrogen, progesterone, cortisol, and other hormones.

And that's where **VNS** may help.

Hormones and the Nervous System: The Missing Link

Your autonomic nervous system (ANS) helps regulate:

- **Hypothalamic-Pituitary-Adrenal (HPA) Axis** → cortisol, DHEA

- **Hypothalamic-Pituitary-Gonadal (HPG) Axis** → estrogen, progesterone, testosterone

- **Ovarian and uterine blood flow** → affected by vagal tone

- **Pain perception** → via brainstem centers like the periaqueductal gray

- **Immune and inflammation levels** → which affect hormone receptor sensitivity

When vagal tone is low—from illness, stress, or inflammation—these systems **lose regulation**, and hormonal symptoms get worse.

Common Hormonal Symptoms in Dysautonomia and Long COVID

Symptom	Vagal/Hormonal Cause
Irregular or missed periods	HPA/HPG axis dysregulation, stress overload
Heavy or painful periods	Loss of parasympathetic uterine control
PMS / PMDD	Mood swings, bloating, low serotonin tied to vagal dysfunction
Anxiety / panic around period	Low progesterone + low vagal tone = no "brake"
Migraines with cycle	Hormonal drop + sympathetic spike
Worsening of POTS or PEM	Estrogen drops → less vascular tone + energy

How VNS May Support Hormonal Health

Effect of VNS	Hormonal Benefit
Activates vagal brake	Calms HPA axis, reduces cortisol spikes
Reduces inflammation	Improves hormone receptor sensitivity
Improves blood flow to pelvis	May ease cramping, PMS, ovarian function
Enhances serotonin & GABA balance	Lifts mood, eases PMDD and anxiety
Modulates hypothalamus–pituitary	Helps rebalance estrogen/progesterone feedback

Some women report **reduced PMS, more regular cycles, and less cycle-related anxiety** after consistent VNS use.

Suggested Timing Around the Menstrual Cycle

Cycle Phase	Suggested VNS Focus
Days 1–5 (menstruation)	Use VNS for cramping, fatigue, and mood
Days 6–14 (follicular)	A calmer phase which is a good time to build tolerance
Days 15–28 (luteal)	Prevent PMS, stabilize mood, avoid sympathetic surge

You may benefit from using **twice-daily sessions during the luteal phase** if that's when symptoms flare.

Research Highlights

- **VNS increases GABA and serotonin**, two calming neurotransmitters often low in PMDD and luteal-phase depression

- Studies in rodents show **vagal stimulation affects ovarian hormone regulation** and fertility outcomes

- **Lower HRV is associated with PMS**, anxiety, and pain—and taVNS improves HRV over time

- In one study, **women with endometriosis** had lower vagal tone and more pain—and vagal activation helped relieve symptoms

How to Support Hormonal Balance Alongside VNS

Support Tool	Why It Helps
Magnesium glycinate	Supports progesterone and muscle relaxation
Omega-3s	Reduces inflammation, stabilizes hormones
Adaptogens *	Gentle cycle support without hormone meds
HRV monitoring +	Detect early stress or sympathetic overdrive
Mindfulness / breathwork	Enhances vagal response and hormone signal stability

* Adaptogens are natural substances—usually herbs, roots, or mushrooms—that help the body adapt to stress and restore balance in key systems, especially the **nervous, immune**, and **endocrine (hormonal)** systems. Unlike stimulants or sedatives that push the body in one direction, adaptogens are thought to "normalize" or *modulate* the body's stress response, whether it's too high or too low. Some examples of adaptogens are Ashwagandha, Reishi Mushroom, Rhodiola, and Holy Basil (Tulsi).

+ HRV stand for Heart Rate Variability and is covered elsewhere in this book.

You don't always need hormones to fix hormones, **sometimes, you need to fix the nerves that regulate them**.

When to Watch Closely

- If your **heart rate drops too much** with VNS during your period, reduce session length
- If symptoms worsen, consider using **lower frequency (15–20 Hz)** during luteal phase
- For women with **low estrogen or amenorrhea**, monitor cycles closely when starting VNS

Summary

Hormones and the nervous system are in constant conversation, and when one is off, the other usually follows.

VNS may help you:

- Smooth out hormone swings
- Ease menstrual pain and anxiety
- Improve cycle regularity
- Regain a sense of inner balance

Your hormones don't exist in a vacuum; they follow the rhythm of your **nervous system**.

And with VNS, you can help reset that rhythm.

VNS for Sleep – Calming the System for Deep, Restorative Rest

How vagus nerve stimulation can help you fall asleep, stay asleep, and wake up refreshed

Sleep is where healing happens: physically, emotionally, hormonally, and neurologically.

But if your vagus nerve is underactive, your body may not **know how to turn off** at night.

Whether it's falling asleep, staying asleep, or waking up exhausted, many Long COVID and dysautonomia patients report that **"sleep doesn't work anymore."**

That's often because their nervous system is stuck in **fight-or-flight**, even at bedtime.

The fix? Shift it back into **rest-and-repair mode**. That's exactly what **vagus nerve stimulation (VNS)** can help do.

Why Sleep Falls Apart in Vagal Dysfunction

To fall asleep, your body needs to:

- Lower sympathetic output (slow down cortisol and norepinephrine)

- Raise parasympathetic (vagal) tone

- Stabilize breathing, digestion, and heart rate

- Sync brainwave patterns into sleep mode

But when vagal tone is low, you stay in **hypervigilance**, and the normal sleep-wake transitions become disrupted.

Signs of Autonomic Sleep Disruption

Sleep Symptom	Possible Vagal Cause
Racing thoughts at night	Low GABA, high sympathetic tone
Difficulty falling asleep	No vagal "brake" on the nervous system
Waking between 1–4am	HPA axis overactivation (stress hormones rising)
Night sweats, HR spikes	Poor vagal modulation of cardiovascular system
Waking unrefreshed	No parasympathetic recovery time during night
Sleep-related gut symptoms	Vagal dysregulation of digestion at night

How VNS Can Improve Sleep Physiology

VNS Effect	Sleep Benefit
Increases parasympathetic tone	Helps initiate and sustain restful states
Decreases cortisol and arousal	Lowers night-time anxiety and early waking

VNS Effect	Sleep Benefit
Improves HRV	Associated with better sleep quality
Modulates respiratory centers	Helps stabilize breathing patterns
Improves serotonin and GABA	Supports deeper sleep architecture (REM, deep sleep)

In studies, taVNS has been shown to **increase slow-wave sleep, reduce sleep latency**, and **improve sleep efficiency**.

Evidence Snapshot

- **taVNS improves HRV** at night, and HRV is a marker of better sleep depth
- Patients using taVNS have shown **reduced sleep onset latency** (fall asleep faster)
- VNS increases **melatonin production** indirectly through brainstem–pineal gland signaling
- One study showed taVNS **improved sleep in PTSD** and **reduced nightmares**

When to Use VNS for Sleep

Time	Reason
30–60 minutes before bed	Allows system to shift into parasympathetic mode
Mid-wake during night	Can help if you wake with HR spike or anxiety
Afternoon only (for sensitive patients)	Use earlier to avoid overstimulation at night

Start with **shorter sessions in the evening** to see how your body responds.

Sample Sleep Protocol

Parameter	Recommended Setting for Sleep
Side	Left ear (tragus or cymba concha)
Frequency	15–20 Hz (lower than usual)
Pulse width	250 µs
Session time	15–30 minutes
Intensity	Mild tingling, no twitching

Use a dim room, calming music, or breathwork while stimulating. Make it a ritual.

Combine VNS with a Sleep Routine

Tool or Habit	Benefit
Magnesium glycinate	Calms nerves, supports melatonin production
Blue-light blockers	Reduces circadian disruption
Weighted blanket	Enhances parasympathetic activation
Gratitude journaling	Improves vagal tone + emotional downshift
Box breathing (4-4-4-4)*	Boosts vagal tone and slows HR before bed

*Details on this breathing technique are in the chapter following the next 'Build a Recovery Routine'

VNS helps create the **internal conditions** that make sleep possible.

Your environment helps reinforce the signal.

What If It Worsens Sleep?

Some users feel more **wired after evening stimulation.** This is usually due to:

- Too high an intensity
- Too close to bedtime
- Overstimulation of cortical areas (especially if using right ear)

Solutions:

- Lower intensity or try **morning use only**
- Use a **calming frequency (15–20 Hz)**
- Add breathwork or light stretching post-session

Summary

Sleep isn't just about melatonin. It's about **nerve signals telling your body it's safe to rest.**

VNS helps send those signals by:

- Shifting your nervous system out of survival mode
- Improving emotional regulation at night
- Calming gut and cardiac activity that disrupts sleep
- Enhancing the natural healing rhythms of deep sleep

You can't force sleep. But with VNS, you can **invite it.**

VNS vs. Other Brain & Nerve Stimulation Therapies

How vagus nerve stimulation stacks up against CES, tDCS, EAT, and trigeminal stimulation

I f you've been exploring non-invasive ways to reset your nervous system, you've probably heard of other tools besides vagus nerve stimulation (VNS):

- **Cranial Electrotherapy Stimulation (CES)**
- **Transcranial Direct Current Stimulation (tDCS)**
- **Trigeminal Nerve Stimulation (TNS)**
- **Epipharyngeal Abrasive Therapy (EAT)**
- **Photobiomodulation (PBM)** and others

Each of these methods **modulates nerve activity**, but they don't all work the same way.

In this chapter, we'll break down how they compare to VNS, when to use them, and how to combine them safely.

What Makes VNS Unique?

Vagus nerve stimulation directly targets the **autonomic nervous system**, the part responsible for:

- Heart rate, digestion, immune control, and inflammation

- Rest, recovery, and emotional regulation
- Hormonal balance and gut-brain communication

It doesn't just calm the brain—it **rebalances the whole-body network** between the brain and the organs.

Feature / Target	VNS	CES	tDCS	TNS	EAT
Primary target	Vagus nerve (autonomic)	Brain electrical activity	Cortical excitability	Trigeminal nerve (sensory/autonomic)	Epipharynx (vagal branches + inflammation)
Main uses	Long COVID, POTS, fatigue, mood, gut issues	Anxiety, insomnia, depression	Depression, fatigue, cognition	ADHD, pain, mood, sleep	Inflammation, fatigue, brain fog
Mechanism	Activates NTS/DMV → modulates vagus output	Alters alpha/beta brain waves	Shifts brain cortex excitability	Affects thalamus, cortex via CN V	Stimulates mucosal vagal endings + reduces cytokines
Anti-inflammatory?	Strong (via CAIP)	Mild (indirect)	Possible (indirect)	Some via limbic deactivation	Local + systemic (via vagus)
HRV improvement?	Yes	Unclear	No direct impact	Variable	Yes (small clinical reports)
Pain reduction?	Moderate	Mild	Moderate	Strong evidence	Yes (headaches, throat pain)
Sleep benefits?	Significant	Commonly used	Some studies	Improves sleep in ADHD	Reduces night symptoms
Device availability	Widely available (taVNS)	Widely available	Research-only or specialty clinics	FDA-cleared for ADHD	Clinical setting only
Side effect risk	Low if used properly	Very low	Mild (tingle, headache)	Low (skin irritation)	Mild (bleeding, discomfort)
Ideal for…	Whole-body dysautonomia, inflammation	Sleep/mood without autonomic reset	Cortical fatigue, brain fog	ADHD, migraine, emotional pain	Chronic inflammation, especially post-viral

Vagus Nerve Stimulation (VNS)

- Best for autonomic dysfunction, inflammation, brain-gut issues

- Improves HRV, fatigue, gut motility, sleep, and immune function
- Easily done at home (taVNS), safe and versatile
- May be **first-line** for Long COVID, POTS, dysautonomia

Cranial Electrotherapy Stimulation (CES)

- Gentle pulses applied to the earlobes or temples
- Alters EEG wave patterns (more alpha = relaxation)
- Strong evidence for **anxiety, insomnia, and stress**
- CES is often used alongside other devices, like the ones listed in the table above: Alpha-Stim, Fisher Wallace, etc.
- Doesn't directly modulate vagal tone or inflammation

Transcranial Direct Current Stimulation (tDCS)

- Direct current passed across scalp to **increase or decrease cortical activity**
- Used for depression, brain fog, post-stroke rehab, and cognitive fatigue
- Helps with **executive function, attention, and motivation**
- Often used in clinics or research settings
- Works best in combination with **mental training tasks**

Trigeminal Nerve Stimulation (TNS)

- Stimulates supraorbital or infraorbital branches of cranial nerve V
- Influences **thalamus, amygdala, and limbic structures**
- Effective for ADHD, depression, PTSD, migraine
- Targets **emotional processing and sensory reactivity**
- Can help regulate heart rate and blood pressure indirectly

Epipharyngeal Abrasive Therapy (EAT)

- Procedure using cotton swabs to stimulate and debride the nasopharynx

- Targets **mucosal inflammation + vagal branches**

- Reduces **cytokines (TNF-α, IL-6, IFN-γ)** and improves fatigue, brain fog

- Shown to **re-balance autonomic tone** (increase HRV)

- Best when done as a **series of weekly treatments** in clinic

When to Choose Each Method

Goal / Symptom	Best Tool(s)
Whole-body dysautonomia, gut, inflammation	EAT + taVNS
Anxiety, insomnia, stress	EAT + CES, taVNS
Depression, cognitive slowness	tDCS, taVNS, TNS + EAT
ADHD, executive dysfunction	TNS, tDCS
Post-COVID inflammation (with sore throat, brain fog)	EAT + taVNS
PTSD, emotional reactivity	taVNS, TNS, CES
PEM, HRV issues, POTS	taVNS, possibly EAT

Can You Combine These Safely?

Yes—in fact, **layering** can be powerful when done strategically:

- **VNS + CES** for anxiety with inflammation

- **VNS + tDCS** for brain fog, executive dysfunction

- **VNS + EAT** for post-viral inflammation and throat-based vagal injury, head pressure, ear fullness, voice changes, swallowing trouble

- **CES at night, VNS in morning** to balance those who are sensitive or easily over-stimulated

- **TNS + VNS** for mood, autonomic issues, and pain syndromes

Together, they form a **powerful toolkit** to retrain your nervous system— gently and consistently.

Don't use multiple devices simultaneously on the **same nerve region** (e.g., both VNS and CES on left ear at the same time). Start with **one**, add the second after assessing response.

Building a Recovery Routine

You've learned how **vagus nerve stimulation (VNS)** and **trigeminal nerve stimulation (TNS)** can reset your nervous system, calm inflammation, and help your brain and body heal from Long COVID.

But here's the truth:

Nerve stimulation works best when it's part of a bigger plan.

This chapter brings it all together. You'll learn how to combine stimulation with key lifestyle strategies—without needing to overhaul your life—so you can get better, faster, and feel better longer.

Why You Need More Than Just a Device

Think of your nervous system like a **garden**. Stimulating the vagus and trigeminal nerves is like watering it—absolutely essential. But if the soil (your body) is full of weeds (inflammation, stress, nutrient deficiencies), your garden won't thrive.

To truly recover, you need:

- A calm nervous system
- Clean fuel (nutrition)
- Movement (even tiny bits)
- Emotional safety and connection
- Rest and repair time

Let's walk through how to layer those on top of your stimulation sessions.

1. Breathing: The Fastest Way to Boost the Vagus Nerve

Slow, deep breathing stimulates the vagus nerve—especially on exhale.

Try this:

Box Breathing (4-4-4-4)

- Inhale 4 seconds
- Hold 4 seconds
- Exhale 4 seconds
- Hold 4 seconds

Do this for 1–3 minutes before or after a stimulation session

Extended Exhale Breathing

- Inhale 4 seconds
- Exhale **6–8 seconds**

This technique especially helps with panic, palpitations, or sleep.

You can do this **anywhere**—in bed, in traffic, or during a flare.

2. Diet: Feeding the Nerves

Your nerves need **clean fuel** and **anti-inflammatory nutrients** to recover. Here's what supports healing:

Nutrient Type	Examples	What It Does
Omega-3 fats	Salmon, sardines, flaxseeds	Lowers brain inflammation
Antioxidants	Berries, greens, turmeric, curcumin	Protects mitochondria and nerves

Nutrient Type	Examples	What It Does
B vitamins	Meat, eggs, leafy greens, methylated B-complex	Supports nerve repair, energy
Magnesium	Pumpkin seeds, spinach, magnesium glycinate	Calms the nervous system
Fermented foods	Sauerkraut, kimchi, kefir	Supports the gut-brain axis

What to reduce:

- **Sugar, alcohol, ultra-processed foods** as they spike inflammation and worsen fatigue
- **Seed oils and fried foods** increase oxidative stress

Even small swaps make a difference—one anti-inflammatory meal at a time.

3. Movement: Gently Rebooting Your System

You don't need intense workouts. In fact, if you have **Post-Exertional Malaise (PEM)**, overdoing it will backfire.

Instead:

Level of Activity	What to Try	How It Helps
Bed-bound	Passive stretching, leg lifts, breathing	Prevents deconditioning

Level of Activity	What to Try	How It Helps
Low energy	Light walks, gentle yoga, tai chi	Boosts circulation and parasympathetic tone
More stable	Swimming, biking, strength training (slow)	Improves mitochondrial and brain function

Pair movement **with breathing and stimulation** for synergistic effects.

4. Emotional Regulation and Social Connection

The vagus nerve is part of your **social engagement system**. That means:

- Facial expressions
- Tone of voice
- Eye contact
- Feeling safe with others

All of this affects—and is affected by—vagal tone.

Simple steps:

- Talk with a calm, trusted friend
- Pet a dog or cat
- Listen to music that moves you
- Laugh or cry during a movie
- Use gentle touch or massage

These aren't "nice extras." They're part of the healing process.

5. Sleep: The Master Reset Button

You won't get better without sleep. Period.

Tips that work best when combined with VNS/TNS:

- Do a **stimulation session before bed**
- Use **blue light blockers** after 8 PM
- Eat your last meal **at least 2 hours before sleep**
- Try **magnesium glycinate** or **taurine**
- Use **box breathing** when falling asleep or waking at night

Track sleep quality over time. You may see better **HRV** (heart rate variability) and deeper rest as the nervous system rebalances.

Sample Recovery Routine

Here's one example of how to put it all together:

Time	Activity
8:00 AM	taVNS (left ear, 25 Hz, 30 min) + breathing
9:00 AM	Walk outside for 10 minutes (sunlight)
12:30 PM	Anti-inflammatory meal (salmon + greens)
3:00 PM	10 min rest + water + deep breathing
6:00 PM	Light stretching or yoga
9:00 PM	TNS session (forehead, 120 Hz, 20 min) + magnesium
10:00 PM	Sleep with blackout curtains + no screens

Even 3–4 of these steps daily can reset your system over time.

Track, Adjust, Repeat

Keep a **simple tracker** for:

- Energy
- Brain fog
- Heart rate
- Sleep quality
- Anxiety/mood

You'll begin to see what's working and when to change things up.

Final Thoughts

You're not just managing symptoms—you're **retraining your nervous system**.

By combining:

- Vagus and trigeminal nerve stimulation
- Gentle lifestyle upgrades
- Nutrition
- Rest
- Breathing

...you give your body the best possible chance to **recover, adapt, and rebuild**.

VNS for POTS – Resetting a Nervous System on Overdrive

How stimulating the vagus nerve can help calm heart rate spikes, dizziness, and fatigue

If you've been diagnosed with **POTS**—or strongly suspect it—you already know how frustrating it is.

You stand up, and your heart races.

You try to function, and you feel dizzy, shaky, tired, nauseous.

Your body feels like it's stuck in overdrive and you can't turn it off.

That's where **vagus nerve stimulation (VNS)** may come in.

This chapter will explain how and why VNS might help, and how to use it safely if you're living with POTS.

What Is POTS, Really?

POTS (Postural Orthostatic Tachycardia Syndrome) is a condition where your heart rate increases too much when you go from lying down to standing up (often 30–50 beats per minute or more).

But it's **not just a heart issue**, it's a **nervous system issue**. More specifically, it's a problem of **autonomic dysregulation**.

The Autonomic Nervous System (ANS) Has Two Sides:

- **Sympathetic ("fight or flight")** – speeds up heart rate, blood pressure, stress

- **Parasympathetic ("rest and digest")** – slows things down, including heart rate

In POTS, the **sympathetic system is stuck "on"** and the vagus nerve (which runs the parasympathetic system) is too weak to counterbalance it.

Where VNS Comes In

Stimulating the vagus nerve—either through the ear (taVNS) or neck — may help **restore this balance**.

What VNS May Improve in POTS:

Symptom / Problem	How VNS May Help
Rapid heart rate (tachycardia)	Increases vagal tone, may slow HR
Dizziness or fainting	Improves blood pressure regulation
Fatigue and brain fog	Boosts cerebral blood flow, lowers inflammation
Nausea, bloating, poor digestion	Enhances vagal control of gut motility
Anxiety and overstimulation	Activates parasympathetic "calming" reflexes
Chronic inflammation	Turns on cholinergic anti-inflammatory pathway (CAIP)

It doesn't cure the root cause of POTS but it **can help modulate the broken signals.**

What the Research Says

There's growing evidence for VNS in autonomic dysfunction, and though POTS-specific research is limited, studies show:

- **taVNS improves heart rate variability (HRV)** – a key sign of better autonomic balance

- VNS can **activate baroreflex sensitivity**, which helps regulate blood pressure and heart rate when you stand

- Patients with **Long COVID–related POTS** have responded well to taVNS in small clinical reports

- A study from *Clinical Autonomic Research* (Baron et al., 2021) noted taVNS may reduce **orthostatic intolerance symptoms**

How to Use VNS for POTS (Safely)

Start with auricular stimulation (taVNS) using the left tragus or cymba concha. Avoid right-side use initially to minimize cardiac effects.

Suggested Protocol:

- **Device**: TENS 7000 or similar unit with adjustable frequency and intensity

- **Electrode**: Double-clip on left ear (tragus or cymba concha)

- **Frequency**: 25 Hz

- **Pulse Width**: 250 µs

- **Duration**: Start with 15–20 minutes, once per day

- **Time of Day**: Morning or midday (avoid bedtime at first if it increases alertness)

Monitor your **heart rate before, during, and after** sessions using a pulse oximeter or wearable device.

Safety Tips

Concern	What to Do
Low heart rate at baseline	Avoid right ear. Start with low intensity, monitor HR.
Pacemaker or arrhythmia	Talk to your doctor before using any form of VNS.
Symptom flare after VNS	Lower session time or pause and try again later.

Always start low and go slow. Some POTS patients are sensitive to even mild interventions.

Combine VNS with Other POTS Tools

VNS works best when paired with **core dysautonomia strategies:**

Strategy	Why It Helps
Hydration + salt	Expands blood volume, prevents crashes
Compression garments	Reduces blood pooling in legs
Pacing + reclined activity	Prevents overexertion + post-exertional crashes
Breathing exercises	Stimulates vagus nerve, lowers sympathetic tone
Mitochondrial support	Reduces fatigue, improves energy production

VNS is the **nervous system signal**. These are the **support systems that make that signal count**.

Signs It May Be Working

You may notice:

- Smaller heart rate increases when standing
- Shorter or milder "crashes"
- Better digestion
- Less anxiety or overstimulation
- Improved HRV score
- Ability to tolerate more activity before symptoms hit

Summary

Vagus nerve stimulation isn't a silver bullet for POTS but it may be one of the **most direct ways** to fix the core issue: a dysregulated nervous system.

- It may lower heart rate, reduce inflammation, and improve vagal tone.
- It's non-invasive, affordable, and adjustable.
- It works best when used **alongside hydration, pacing, and lifestyle strategies.**
- Start cautiously and **track your response** over time.

Epipharyngeal Abrasive Therapy (EAT): A Gentle Reset for Vagus and Trigeminal Nerves

O ne of the most overlooked, yet powerful tools in vagus and trigeminal nerve rehabilitation is something called **Epipharyngeal Abrasive Therapy**, or **EAT**. While it may sound intimidating, this technique is actually a **simple, non-invasive procedure** that works on a powerful reflex hub deep in the back of your nose and upper throat—an area that connects directly to both the **vagus** and **trigeminal nerves**.

Let's break it down and show you how EAT might help with symptoms like **brain fog, dizziness, fatigue, chronic cough, postnasal drip**, and even **insomnia**—especially in Long COVID.

What Is EAT?

EAT involves gently rubbing a cotton-tipped swab against the back of your upper throat and nasal passage—specifically the area known as the **epipharynx**. This area isn't a well-defined anatomical structure, but it's essentially the region above your soft palate and behind your nasal cavity.

A trained provider performs the procedure using a **small camera (endoscope)** to guide the swab. The mucosa (mucus membrane) is numbed with **lidocaine spray**, so the treatment is painless, and most people don't gag at all.

Please don't try this at home—it requires precision and visualization of the area, especially near the **openings of the Eustachian tubes**.

Why Stimulate the Epipharynx?

The upper throat and back of the nasal cavity are **densely innervated by vagus and trigeminal nerve endings**. When this area becomes chronically inflamed—as it often does in **Long COVID, chronic sinus issues, or viral infections**—it can **send the wrong signals to the brain**, keeping the nervous system stuck in an inflamed, overactive state.

EAT stimulates the nerves directly while also helping reduce local inflammation, which may improve symptoms throughout the body.

How Does EAT Work?

EAT is believed to help in several ways:

- **Stimulates vagus nerve endings** in the throat and nasopharynx
- **Reduces inflammatory signals**, including cytokines like TNF-alpha and IL-1
- **Improves drainage** of the lymphatic tissue behind the nose
- **Reduces swelling** and irritation in nearby nerve clusters
- **Interrupts chronic signaling loops** that may keep the nervous system on "high alert"

Over time, as inflammation reduces, the treated tissue **bleeds less**, and patients often notice steady improvement in symptoms.

What Symptoms Can EAT Improve?

EAT has been reported to improve a **wide range of symptoms**, particularly in patients with **Long COVID, ME/CFS, or upper respiratory inflammation**:

- Postnasal drip and runny nose
- Throat irritation, chronic cough, hoarseness

- Nasal congestion or chronic sinus pressure

- Eustachian tube dysfunction, ear fullness, tinnitus

- Dizziness, vertigo, lightheadedness

- Headaches and facial pressure

- Snoring, poor sleep, daytime fatigue

- Brain fog and low mood

- Acid reflux, heartburn

- Fatigue that feels neurological, not just physical

Why It's Especially Relevant in Long COVID

Many Long COVID patients unknowingly suffer from **chronic inflammation in the upper throat and nasal cavity**—called **epipharyngitis**. This inflammation doesn't always cause pain, but it can constantly stimulate nerves like the **vagus** and **trigeminal**, causing symptoms across multiple systems: neurological, digestive, cardiovascular, and more.

EAT acts like a **reset button** for this overstimulated system. It doesn't solve everything—but when added to a larger treatment plan, it can move the needle in a way that few therapies can.

Case Study: EAT in a Patient With Long COVID, Brain Fog, and Dizziness

Patient Profile

Name: Sarah M. (pseudonym)

Age: 38

History: Previously healthy, active woman who developed Long COVID symptoms 3 months after an acute COVID-19 infection. Her initial infection was mild, with no hospitalization. She never fully recovered.

Presenting Symptoms

- **Persistent brain fog**, described as "walking through molasses"
- **Daily dizziness**, especially when standing quickly or turning her head
- **Chronic throat clearing and postnasal drip**
- **Tinnitus** in the right ear and fullness in both ears
- **Unrefreshing sleep and daytime fatigue**
- Mild **orthostatic intolerance**, worsened with activity or stress

Evaluation

Routine bloodwork and brain imaging were normal. Vitals revealed a slight postural heart rate increase (consistent with POTS), but no overt cardiac disease.

Notably, nasoendoscopic evaluation revealed **chronic epipharyngitis**: reddened, congested mucosa in the **epipharyngeal area** with visible pooling of mucus.

Intervention: Epipharyngeal Abrasive Therapy (EAT)

- Sarah underwent her **first EAT session** using topical lidocaine and a flexible endoscope (camera).
- A cotton swab was used to gently abrade the epipharyngeal mucosa and around the **Eustachian tube orifices**.
- She tolerated the procedure well. No bleeding during the first session. Mild post-procedural soreness for 12 hours.

Clinical Response

Session	Notable Changes
After 1st session	Improved clarity of thought for ~24 hours; ears felt less "clogged"
After 3rd session	Significant reduction in postnasal drip and daily dizziness; brain fog less frequent
After 6th session	Reported "first full night of restful sleep in over a year"; resumed light exercise
After 8 sessions	Tinnitus no longer constant; fatigue improved ~40% from baseline
Post-treatment	Now receives maintenance EAT once per month along with vagus nerve stimulation and adrenal support

Takeaway

Sarah's case highlights how **chronic epipharyngitis can silently drive neurological and autonomic symptoms** by persistently stimulating the **vagus and trigeminal nerves**. EAT helped **break the inflammatory feedback loop**, allowing her nervous system to reset and begin healing. Repetition and consistency is the key to success with the EAT procedures. One procedure is typically not enough.

Final Thoughts

EAT is a **low-risk, high-impact** therapy that directly targets the **neuroinflammatory loop** keeping many chronic symptoms alive. By stimulating vagus and trigeminal nerve branches where they're most exposed—and often inflamed—it helps **calm the system**, reduce symptoms, and support healing from the top down.

If you're struggling with post-COVID symptoms, unexplained fatigue, or stubborn sinus and ear issues, **ask your provider about EAT**. It may be the missing piece of your recovery puzzle.

Real People, Real Healing

How vagus and trigeminal nerve stimulation helped others reclaim their lives from Long COVID.

You've made it through the science. You've learned the methods. But sometimes what we need most is **hope**—and **proof** that recovery is possible. I have seen it work, over and over.

This chapter shares stories from real patients who used **nerve stimulation**—along with simple lifestyle changes—to fight back against Long COVID.

Each story shows what worked, what didn't, and how long it took to see results.

Case 1: "I Couldn't Even Walk to the Mailbox"

Name: Amanda

Age: 37

Main symptoms: Extreme fatigue, dizziness, PEM, brain fog

Start of Long COVID: November 2021

"Before COVID, I was running 5Ks. A month after getting sick, I could barely make it from my bedroom to the kitchen. My heart would race, and I felt like I had the flu every day."

Amanda started with **auricular vagus nerve stimulation (taVNS)** using a TENS 7000 and an ear clip, once daily for 30 minutes.

After 3 weeks:

- Energy crashes became less severe
- Brain fog slightly improved

After 6 weeks:

- She could walk around the block without triggering PEM
- Started adding short breathing sessions before taVNS

"It felt slow, but every week I was just a little more 'me.' By month three, I was doing yoga again."

Case 2: "Brain Fog Was Ruining My Job"

Name: Mike

Age: 42

Main symptoms: Brain fog, focus problems, word-finding issues

Start of Long COVID: February 2022

Mike works in IT and found himself staring at screens without knowing what he was doing. He tried supplements and dietary changes, but they didn't help much.

He added **trigeminal nerve stimulation (TNS)** using forehead pads and a TENS unit:

- 120 Hz
- 250 µs pulse width
- 30 minutes each evening

After 10 days:

- He noticed clearer thinking in the mornings
- His wife noticed he was less irritable

After 1 month:

- Able to concentrate for hours at a time
- Started pairing stimulation with morning taVNS for added benefit

"This combo saved my career. It brought my brain back online."

Case 3: "I Had POTS. Now I Can Stand Without Passing Out."

Name: Elaine

Age: 55

Main symptoms: POTS (Postural Orthostatic Tachycardia Syndrome), nausea, fatigue

Start of Long COVID: July 2020

Elaine had seen 5 doctors and was told to "stay hydrated." Her heart rate would spike from 70 to 130 just from standing up. She started taVNS in 2022 under clinical guidance.

Her protocol:

- taVNS (left tragus, 25 Hz, 250 µs, 30 min twice a day)
- Pyridostigmine 30 mg once daily
- Gentle walking and breathing

After 2 weeks:

- Resting HR stabilized
- Less dizziness with posture changes

After 6 weeks:

- Heart rate would only rise to 95 with standing
- Resumed gardening and short trips outside

"It's not just the nerve stim. It's what you pair it with. For me, it was fluids, meds, and time."

Case 4: "My Son Got His Focus Back"

Name: Ethan (with mom, Rachel)

Age: 10

Main symptoms: ADHD-like symptoms after COVID: distraction, irritability, poor sleep

Ethan had never had behavioral issues before getting COVID. Afterward, his teachers noticed trouble focusing and emotional swings.

Rachel started him on **Monarch eTNS**, a device approved for pediatric ADHD.

Routine:

- 1 hour per night while asleep
- Started in week 3 of post-COVID recovery

After 3 weeks:

- Sleep improved
- Fewer meltdowns

After 6 weeks:

- Teacher reported better classroom behavior
- Ethan said, "I feel like my brain isn't so loud anymore."

"As a parent, it was a lifesaver. We weren't looking for a miracle; we just wanted our son back."

Case 5: "As a Doctor, I Needed Something Evidence-Based"

Name: Dr. H

Age: 49

Main symptoms: Burnout, fatigue, unexplained inflammation after COVID exposure

Profession: Anesthesiologist

Dr. H wasn't convinced at first. He looked into the science behind the cholinergic anti-inflammatory pathway and decided to try taVNS.

Protocol:

- taVNS (TENS unit + tragus clip)
- Twice daily, 25 Hz
- Paired with cold showers and intermittent fasting

After 2 weeks:

- CRP dropped
- Mood lifted

After 1 month:

- Returned to full work schedule
- Added red light therapy + NAD+ boosters

"The science was sound. Once I felt it working, I realized I wasn't just coping anymore—I was recovering."

What These Stories Show

Every recovery is different. But the patterns are clear:

Pattern Observed	What It Means
Progress takes **weeks, not days**	Be consistent—it's retraining, not instant relief
Combining **multiple therapies works**	VNS/TNS + movement + nutrition = better results
You can start **at any severity level**	Even bedbound patients made progress
Recovery is **nonlinear**	Expect good days and bad—don't quit after one setback

Your Story Could Be Next

You don't need to do this alone. There's a growing community of patients and providers using **neuromodulation** to treat Long COVID—and sharing what works.

Keep tracking, keep adapting, and keep going.

Rewiring the System: How Your Nervous System Learns to Heal

You've seen how vagus and trigeminal nerve stimulation can calm inflammation, regulate heart rate, and clear brain fog. But here's the deeper magic:

Your brain and nervous system can *change* —physically and functionally— in response to these inputs.

This ability is called **neuroplasticity**. And it's the reason why nerve stimulation doesn't just "mask symptoms." It helps **rewire the system** so you can **stay better** over time.

What Is Neuroplasticity?

Neuroplasticity means your brain and nervous system are adaptable, like soft clay. They can:

- **Form new connections**

- **Strengthen or weaken old ones**

- **Recover lost functions**

- **Learn new ways of responding**

This happens all the time—during learning, recovery from injury, or even emotional healing. But it works best when the nervous system is **stable and supported** which is exactly what vagus and trigeminal nerve stimulation provide.

How Vagus and Trigeminal Stimulation Use Neuroplasticity

When you apply electrical stimulation to your vagus or trigeminal nerves, you're not just flipping a switch.

You're **training your nervous system**, like physical therapy for your brain.

Here's how it works:

Stimulation Type	Neuroplastic Effect
taVNS	Activates the nucleus tractus solitarius (NTS) which regulates inflammation, improves autonomic tone
TNS	Stimulates sensory pathways which improve cortical focus, mood circuits, and attention systems
Repeated use	Builds stronger, more stable circuits for calm, focus, digestion, and energy
Long-term use	Rewires threat responses which means less overreaction to stress, pain, or fatigue triggers

These changes don't happen overnight. But with **consistent input**, the brain begins to re-route traffic away from broken pathways and toward healing ones.

Example: From Crash to Calm

Let's say you have **Long COVID dysautonomia**:

- Your heart races when you stand.

- Your digestion is sluggish.

- You feel anxious for no reason.

This is a **"stuck" stress pattern**—a feedback loop. Your nervous system thinks it's in danger and keeps reacting.

With **daily stimulation**, over time:

1. You activate the vagus or trigeminal nerve.

2. That calms the brainstem and quiets danger signals.

3. Your heart rate, gut, and stress hormones start to rebalance.

4. Your brain forms **new patterns** of regulation.

5. Eventually, your body does this **on its own**, with less and less need for stimulation.

That's **neuroplasticity** at work: you go from reactivity to resilience.

What Helps (or Hurts) Neuroplasticity

Things That Enhance Neuroplasticity

Boosts Healing	Why It Works
Sleep	Brain rewires most during deep sleep
Breathwork	Increases parasympathetic tone
Moderate movement	Stimulates blood flow and BDNF (brain fertilizer)
Anti-inflammatory diet	Supports brain repair at a cellular level
TNS + taVNS + consistency	Daily input creates new default settings

Things That Block It

Slows or Stops Progress	Why It Hurts
Chronic stress	Keeps brain in fight-or-flight mode
Inflammation	Disrupts neuro-signaling and tissue repair
Sedentary lifestyle	Reduces brain oxygen and nerve stimulation
Sleep deprivation	Disrupts memory and repair pathways
Giving up too soon	No consistent signal = no change

How Long Does It Take?

That depends on:

- The severity of your dysfunction
- How consistent your practice is
- What other supports (diet, movement, sleep) you've added

But on average:

Time Frame	Expected Changes
Week 1–2	Slight improvements (energy, sleep, mood)
Week 3–5	Stronger HRV, reduced symptom severity
Week 6–8	Noticeable shifts in cognitive clarity, resilience
Week 12+	Deeper baseline recovery; fewer crashes

Neuroplasticity is **slow but permanent**, the longer you keep it up, the stronger your recovery becomes.

Why Your Nervous System Needs Repetition

Repetition tells your brain:

"This is the new normal. Let's build around it."

That's why you don't need to crank the intensity of stimulation higher and higher. You just need **daily nudges**.

Think of it like learning to walk again, you don't need to sprint, you just need to **take the same steps, every day**, until your system takes over.

Takeaway: Train It to Heal It

- Vagus and trigeminal nerve stimulation are **training tools** for your nervous system

- You're helping it **remember how to stay calm, digest food, regulate heart rate, and think clearly**

- Recovery happens through **neuroplasticity**, not overnight, but over time

- What you do consistently shapes your outcome

Your nervous system is listening—give it the right signals, and it can learn to heal.

Advanced Tools to Boost Nerve Recovery

What if you could accelerate nerve healing with the right environment?

By now, you've learned how vagus and trigeminal nerve stimulation can shift your nervous system back into balance. But if you want to go further—or if your symptoms have plateaued—there are **additional therapies** that can help push recovery forward.

These advanced techniques work by activating your body's natural repair systems:

- Nerve regeneration
- Mitochondrial repair
- Anti-inflammatory signaling
- Stress adaptation (hormesis)

Let's break down the safest, most effective ones you can try at home or with guidance.

1. Cold Exposure

Harnessing the power of cold to calm inflammation and reset stress responses

Cold exposure (like ice baths or cold showers) activates the **vagus nerve** and stimulates a process called **hormesis** (a controlled stress that leads to greater resilience).

Benefits:

- Increases **parasympathetic tone**

- Boosts **mitochondrial function**

- Reduces **inflammatory cytokines**

- Helps control **heart rate and breathing**

How to Do It Safely:

Method	Duration	Notes
Cold face splash	10–20 seconds	Easiest starter; good vagus activation
Cold shower (30–60°F)	30–90 seconds daily	End shower cold or alternate hot/cold
Ice bath (if tolerated)	1–3 minutes max	Only with supervision or proper prep

Start slowly and always breathe deeply. **Never push through shivering or panic.**

2. Red Light Therapy (Photobiomodulation)

Giving your mitochondria the fuel to repair and recharge

Red light and **near-infrared light** can penetrate your skin and stimulate healing in the cells, especially the mitochondria that power nerves.

How It Works:

- Activates **cytochrome c oxidase** which boosts ATP

- Reduces **oxidative stress**

- Increases **nerve growth factor (NGF)**
- Supports **mitochondrial biogenesis** (making new mitochondria)

What It Helps:

- Brain fog, fatigue
- Nerve pain or tingling
- Slow healing
- Post-COVID mitochondrial dysfunction

At-Home Use:

Light Type	Wavelengths (nm)	Application Area	Frequency
Red light	630–660 nm	Skin, face, neck	5–10 min, daily
Near-infrared (NIR)	800–850 nm	Penetrates deeper	Chest, head, gut
Full-body panels	Combo (660+850)	Whole-body benefit	10–20 min, 3–5x/week

Always follow safety precautions (no direct eye exposure unless using eyewear).

3. Supporting Nerve Regeneration

Nutrients, tools, and habits that help nerves rebuild

Nerves take time to heal—but you can help them regenerate faster with key nutrients and practices:

Key Nutrients for Nerve Repair:

Nutrient	Function	Food/Supplement Sources
Vitamin B1 (Benfotiamine)	Repairs myelin, reduces nerve pain	Pork, sunflower seeds, supplements
Vitamin B12 (Methylcobalamin)	Builds nerve sheaths, improves transmission	Meat, eggs, sublingual B12
Omega-3s (DHA/EPA)	Supports nerve structure, reduces inflammation	Fish oil, algae oil
Alpha-lipoic acid (ALA)	Antioxidant; reduces nerve sensitivity	Supplement (R-ALA form preferred)
Acetyl-L-carnitine (ALCAR)	Enhances mitochondrial and nerve repair	Supplement (500–1000 mg/day)
Magnesium	Calms nerve excitability	Magnesium glycinate, citrate

Bonus Tools:

- **TENS therapy on affected areas**: Can help nerve firing patterns
- **Moderate activity**: Keeps blood flowing to nerve-rich areas
- **Fascial release or gentle massage**: Helps loosen nerve pathways

What About Peptides or Prescription Tools?

Emerging therapies include:

- **BDNF boosters** (Brain-Derived Neurotrophic Factor): such as lion's mane mushroom

- **Peptides** like BPC-157 or Semax (clinical guidance only)

- **Low-dose Naltrexone (LDN)**: Calms microglial activation in the brain

- **Hyperbaric Oxygen Therapy (HBOT)**: Repairs damaged tissue via oxygenation (especially useful post-COVID but requires clinical access)

These advanced therapies are promising but should be used with **medical oversight**—especially if you're already using VNS/TNS.

Stack It—Don't Stress It

You don't need to do everything at once. Try **stacking** stimulation with one advanced therapy at a time:

- Do **taVNS after a red light session**

- Add **cold face splashes before bed**

- Take **ALA or omega-3s with breakfast**

- Use **magnesium at night** to support repair during sleep

Small, repeated nudges = lasting change.

Final Takeaway

- These advanced tools **support nerve regeneration**, calm inflammation, and improve energy.

- Start slowly, track how you respond, and stay consistent.

- These are not shortcuts but **accelerators**, when they're used alongside core strategies like VNS, TNS, movement, sleep, and nutrition.

Stuck? Here's How to Get Unstuck

When nerve stimulation doesn't seem to be working, here's what to check, change, or troubleshoot.

You've done the work: the stimulation sessions, the breathing, the supplements. Maybe you've even tried red light or cold exposure. But what if you're **not improving** or your symptoms come roaring back?

The truth is: **recovery isn't always a straight line**. In this chapter, you'll learn what to do when you hit a plateau, crash, or don't feel any difference—yet.

Step 1: Revisit Your Stimulation Setup

Let's rule out technical issues first.

Common Mistakes:

Problem	What to Try Instead
Wrong ear placement (for taVNS)	Use the **tragus** or **cymba concha**, not the earlobe

Problem	What to Try Instead
Intensity too low or too high	You should feel a gentle **tingling**, not pain or nothing
Only using 1 electrode	You need a **complete circuit**—both leads must be attached unless you are using a double-contact clip
Wrong frequency or pulse width	Try **25 Hz, 250 μs** for taVNS; **120 Hz** for TNS
Inconsistent usage	Daily sessions are ideal; 1–2x per day for best effect

Make sure your device is capable of custom settings. Many cheap EMS units **don't allow** proper taVNS programming.

Step 2: Check for Overstimulation

Yes, you *can* do too much. Signs include:

- Fatigue after stimulation

- Racing heart or dizziness (especially with **right-ear** use)

- Muscle twitching or pain at electrode site

What to Do:

- **Back off the intensity** by lowering the mA setting

- Use **left ear only**

- Cut session time to **15–20 minutes**

- Skip a day and resume gently

Start low, go slow. Think of it like physical therapy—don't overtrain your nerves.

Step 3: Address Nervous System "Blockers"

Sometimes stimulation can't work well until bigger issues are cleared.

Look for:

Blocker Type	What It Does	What Helps
Ongoing inflammation	Interferes with nerve signaling	Anti-inflammatory diet, omega-3s, sleep
Gut dysbiosis	Impairs vagus–brain connection	Probiotics, low histamine diet
Unmanaged stress/trauma	Keeps system in fight-or-flight	Gentle somatic work, vagal breathing
Sleep deprivation	Shuts down neuroplasticity	Prioritize sleep routine and magnesium
Mold, Lyme, toxins	Act as constant irritants	Test + treat root causes with a provider

If your system is "jammed," stimulation may need to be paused until you remove the interference.

Step 4: Switch It Up

If you've been doing the same thing for weeks with no change, it's okay to experiment.

Try:

- **Right ear stimulation** (carefully, check HR during session)
- Switching from **TENS ear clip to sticky electrodes**

- Using **TNS instead of taVNS** (or vice versa)

- Changing **frequency** slightly day-to-day (e.g., 25 Hz → 21 Hz → 27 Hz)

- Doing **stimulation in the morning** instead of evening (or both)

These changes may help **avoid nervous system habituation** (where the brain tunes out the signal).

Step 5: Track Symptoms Objectively

Sometimes we *are* improving—just not noticing.

Try a simple daily log:

Date	Energy (0–10)	Brain Fog	HR on standing	Sleep Quality	Notes
Day 1	3	7	110 → 140 bpm	Poor	Started taVNS
Day 7	5	5	110 → 125 bpm	Fair	Added red light

This helps detect patterns, slow gains, and triggers.

Step 6: Get Professional Support

If you're still stuck after 6–8 weeks:

- Work with a **Long COVID-literate provider**

- Consider deeper testing: cortisol, HRV, gut health, micronutrients

- Ask about adding therapies like:

  o Low-dose naltrexone (LDN)

141

- o Acetylcholinesterase inhibitors (e.g., pyridostigmine)

- o Mitochondrial support (e.g., CoQ10, NAD+)

Even the best tools sometimes need the right guidance to shine.

Reminder: Progress Can Look Messy

Recovery might look like:

- Two steps forward, one back

- A random crash after a good week

- Feeling better mentally but still tired physically

That's normal. The nervous system is complex, but it's also **forgiving and trainable**.

Final Takeaway

If stimulation isn't working yet:

- **Double-check your settings**

- **Avoid overstimulation**

- **Look for other roadblocks**

- **Switch it up strategically**

- **Track your progress**

- **Seek help if needed**

You're not doing something wrong. You're just learning what your body needs—and that's the most powerful step of all.

Your Recovery Roadmap

How to build real progress, one month at a time

You've got the tools. You've learned how stimulation works. You've even seen what to do when things stall.

Now it's time to **put it all together**.

This chapter gives you a **clear 3-month plan** for using vagus and trigeminal nerve stimulation—alongside lifestyle changes—to maximize recovery from Long COVID, dysautonomia, or lingering post-viral symptoms.

No guessing. No overwhelm. Just a simple structure to follow, adapt, and grow with.

Why a Month-by-Month Plan?

Because your nervous system doesn't heal all at once—it responds to **repetition and layering**. Each month has a focus:

- **Month 1:** Reset your baseline

- **Month 2:** Build momentum

- **Month 3:** Stabilize and adapt

Month 1: Reset the Nervous System

Main goal: Calm inflammation and reestablish autonomic balance

What You're Doing:

- **taVNS** (left tragus, 25 Hz, 250 μs) – once daily, 30 minutes
- **Box breathing** or extended exhale – daily for 15 minutes
- **Anti-inflammatory nutrition** – fewer sugars, more omega-3s and veggies
- **Sleep hygiene** – regular bedtime, no blue light before bed. This includes computer screens, TV, and smart phones. If you must use them, use a blue light filter program available on most electrical appliances.
- **Light movement** – gentle stretching, walks, or just sitting upright if bedbound

Weekly Milestones:

Week	Focus	Notes
1	Learn stimulation setup	Test placement, intensity, and timing
2	Add breathing + sleep support	Magnesium, wind-down routine before bedtime
3	Start nutrition cleanup	Add omega-3s and hydrate more
4	Consistency over perfection	Stick to once-daily stim + gentle walks

What to expect: Slight changes in energy, mood, heart rate, or digestion. Sleep might improve first.

Month 2: Build Recovery Momentum

Main goal: Strengthen brain-body signaling and stabilize energy

What You're Adding:

- **Trigeminal Nerve Stimulation (TNS)** – 120 Hz, 20–30 minutes in the evening

- **taVNS frequency rotation** – shift between 21–27 Hz every few days

- **More movement** – standing stretches, yoga, or brief walks if tolerated

- **Red light therapy** (optional) – 5–10 min near face/neck/abdomen, 3–5x/week

- **Track symptoms** – HR, fatigue, fog, sleep, mood

Weekly Milestones:

Week	Focus	Notes
5	Introduce TNS or red light	Use forehead pads for 20–30 min at night
6	Add tracking journal	Log HR, brain fog, sleep, mood
7	Adjust stimulation based on response	Increase duration or switch sides
8	Combine modalities	Try stim + breath + light combo

What to expect:

- More stable mornings
- Less crashing from light activity
- Brain fog lifts in small windows

Month 3: Stabilize and Expand

Main goal: Rebuild resilience, expand capacity, and taper dependence

What You're Fine-Tuning:

- Try **2 stim sessions/day**: morning taVNS + evening TNS
- Gradually **increase physical tolerance**: 5–15 min of movement
- Add **cognitive work**: memory games, reading, socializing
- Integrate **cold exposure** or **HBOT** if accessible
- Reassess supplements: B12, ALA, NAD+, CoQ10

Weekly Milestones:

Week	Focus	Notes
9	Try 2x/day stimulation	AM (taVNS) + PM (TNS) or alternate ears
10	Add mild stress (cold, standing tasks)	Test your new baseline
11	Track best-response patterns	Which stim setting/time gives best result
12	Evaluate next phase (continue or taper)	Are you ready to reduce frequency?

What to expect:

- Clearer energy patterns
- Better post-exertional tolerance
- More independence from daily stimulation (some taper to every other day)

What If You Need a Slower Plan?

Then take 2–3 weeks per milestone instead of 1. This is your journey.

After Month 3: What's Next?

Situation	What to Do
Feeling 70–90% better	Taper stimulation to every other day, then weekly
Still symptomatic	Repeat Month 2 until stable, then reassess
Still crashing or flaring	Pause stim; focus on sleep, gut, and inflammation
Mostly mental symptoms	Emphasize TNS, light cognitive rehab, red light
New symptoms show up	Rule out mold, infections, cortisol issues

Recovery takes time, but your **system is trainable**. This plan gives it the consistency, inputs, and safety to rewire at its own pace.

Final Thoughts

- Nerve stimulation isn't a quick fix—it's a **retraining protocol.**
- Paired with the right lifestyle changes, it can reprogram the very systems that broke down.
- The body is not broken, it's **adaptive.**
- With daily signals, it can remember how to heal.

Build Your Own Nerve Healing Plan

Not every body is the same—here's how to create a recovery plan that fits you.

You've now got a full toolbox:

- Vagus nerve stimulation (taVNS)
- Trigeminal nerve stimulation (TNS)
- Red light therapy
- Breathing, cold, and supplements
- Tracking, pacing, and lifestyle changes

But here's the reality: **You don't need every tool all the time.** What matters most is **what works for your nervous system**—and what symptoms you're trying to fix.

This chapter walks you through how to **customize your own protocol**.

Start with Your Symptom Profile

Use this chart to identify your most bothersome symptoms and match them with best-fit tools:

Symptom / Condition	Best Starting Tools
Brain fog, cognitive fatigue	TNS (evening), taVNS (morning), red light (forehead)
Anxiety or panic	taVNS (left ear), breathwork, magnesium
Palpitations / high HR / POTS	taVNS (left only), hydration, pacing, compression
Fatigue / crashes after activity	taVNS, mitochondrial support, red light
Poor sleep / waking at night	TNS (evening), taVNS post-dinner, box breathing
Low mood or depression	TNS (AM), taVNS (midday), cold exposure
GI symptoms (nausea, IBS, reflux)	taVNS (left ear), breathing, ST36 acupuncture point
Inflammation / joint pain	taVNS, omega-3s, ALA, red light

Device + Dose Matching Guide

Pick the right device and setup for your symptoms:

Tool	Best Use Case	Frequency	Duration
taVNS	Inflammation, HRV, digestion, fatigue	Daily (1–2x/day)	30 min (left ear)
TNS	Focus, mood, insomnia, brain fog	Evening or bedtime	20–30 min
Red light (660/850 nm)	Mito support, pain, cognitive energy	3–5x/week	10–15 min
Cold exposure	Anxiety, HR control, morning reset	3–4x/week	30–90 sec
Breathing	Stress, vagal tone, PEM flare support	1–3x/day	5 min

Timing Tips Based on Your Needs

Goal	Best Time for Stim/Tool Use
Boost alertness or brain clarity	AM taVNS + red light + water
Calm racing heart or anxiety	taVNS + box breathing (midday)
Prevent evening PEM crash	2nd taVNS session at 3–5 PM
Improve sleep quality	TNS before bed + magnesium
Support digestion / motility	taVNS 30 min after meals
Recover after stress or flare	Cold face splash + taVNS + rest

Fine-Tuning Based on Your Reaction

If You Feel...	Try This Adjustment
No sensation during stim	Wet clip, try different electrode position
Too stimulated / jittery	Lower intensity, switch to AM-only use
No change after 3 weeks	Add TNS, try 2x/day, or rotate frequency
Dizzy with right ear stim	Stop right ear use; switch to left only
Improvement, then plateau	Add red light, supplements, or pacing tweaks

Sample Custom Protocols

Mild Brain Fog + Anxiety

- AM: taVNS (left tragus, 25 Hz, 30 min)
- PM: TNS (forehead, 120 Hz, 20 min)
- Daily: 5 min box breathing + omega-3s

PEM + POTS

- AM: taVNS + compression socks + salt + electrolytes
- PM: Light movement → red light → taVNS again
- Daily: Pacing chart + magnesium at night

GI Symptoms + Low Mood

- After meals: taVNS (left ear, 25 Hz, 30 min)
- Afternoon: red light (abdomen)
- Evening: TNS + low histamine diet + probiotics

When to Reassess

Revisit your plan every **3–4 weeks**:

Sign You Should Adjust	What to Change
No change in main symptom	Switch frequency or add second tool
Energy improving but crashing	Add pacing protocol or recheck PEM triggers
Better mood, still brain fog	Add red light or NAD+ supplement
Side effects (HR, dizziness)	Lower dose or reduce frequency

Final Words on Personalization

There's no one-size-fits-all recovery. But that's a good thing.

Because once you learn to listen to your nervous system—and give it the **right signal at the right time**—you unlock your own healing path.

Start small

Track responses

Adjust as needed

Stay consistent

This is how healing happens.

HRV – How to Know If You're Healing

Your heart's rhythm can tell you how well your nervous system is working and recovering.

You may have heard of **heart rate variability**, or **HRV**, and wondered what it means—or whether you should even pay attention to it.

The short answer is: **yes, you should**.

HRV is one of the **best non-invasive markers** of nervous system health, vagal tone, and recovery. It's not just a number, it's a **real-time report card** on how your brain, body, and stress response systems are doing.

And when you're using vagus or trigeminal nerve stimulation, **HRV can tell you if it's working.**

What Is HRV, Really?

Your heart doesn't beat like a metronome. Instead, the time between each beat changes slightly—and that's **a good thing**.

For example:

- One beat: 1.00 seconds apart
- Next beat: 0.92 seconds
- Next: 1.08 seconds

This is **heart rate variability**—a flexible, adaptable rhythm. It means your nervous system is **able to respond to and recover** from challenges.

Low HRV = stiff, stressed system

High HRV = calm, resilient system

HRV and the Vagus Nerve

HRV is mainly controlled by the **vagus nerve**, especially the **parasympathetic branch** (the "rest and repair" side).

That means:

- More vagal activity → higher HRV
- Overactive stress response → lower HRV
- Recovery → gradual rise in HRV

When you use **taVNS or TNS**, your HRV should eventually **go up**—that's a sign your nervous system is healing.

Why HRV Is So Useful

HRV can help you:

- **Track your recovery** over time
- **Spot a crash or flare** before it happens
- **Test what helps you** (or hurts you)
- **Time your activity** and stimulation
- Stay motivated with **real, objective feedback**

You're not just guessing anymore; you're **watching your nervous system in action**.

How to Measure HRV

Because there is more than one way to calculate HRV, it is important that you are comparing apples to apples. The most common two metrics are RMSSD and SDNN.

Tool	Metric Measured	Notes
Oura Ring	RMSSD (Root Mean Square of Successive Differences)	Best for overnight HRV and daily readiness score (parasympathetic tone)
Whoop Strap	RMSSD	Focuses on recovery, strain, and sleep performance via HRV
Apple Watch	SDNN (Standard Deviation of NN intervals)	Measures during rest or Breathe app sessions; not ideal for continuous tracking
Polar / Garmin Chest Strap	R-R Intervals (raw data for RMSSD/SDNN)	Best for live, high-resolution HRV tracking during exercise or rest
Garmin Smartwatches	RMSSD-derived (reported as "Stress" or HRV status)	HRV measured during sleep or rest, interpreted via stress/recovery metrics
Fitbit (Sense, Charge 5+)	RMSSD (overnight)	Tracks HRV during sleep; shown as trends, not live measurements

If possible, use the **same time of day** and **same device** for consistency.

HRV Metrics to Know

HRV Metric	What It Means	Values
RMSSD	Reflects parasympathetic (vagal) activity	**25–65 ms** (younger healthy adults often 40–65 ms; < 20 ms suggests low vagal tone)
SDNN	Total variability (affected by all systems)	**> 50 ms = healthy**, 20–50 ms = reduced, < 20 ms = very low (based on 24-hour recordings)
LF/HF ratio	Balance between sympathetic and parasympathetic	**0.5 – 2.0** is considered balanced; > 2.0 indicates sympathetic dominance, < 0.5 indicates parasympathetic dominance
Baseline HRV	Your personal average (not just "high or low")	

For most home users, **RMSSD** or the "HRV Score" your device gives you is enough.

What's a Good HRV?

There's no universal "good" number—**what matters is your trend.** Your HRV should gradually **increase or stabilize** as you recover.

Typical RMSSD ranges:

- 20–30 ms = low vagal tone

- 40–60 ms = moderate

- 70+ ms = excellent resilience

But your best number is your own baseline. Don't compare to others—compare to your own HRV history.

What Affects HRV?

Improves HRV	Lowers HRV
taVNS / TNS	Infections or inflammation
Good sleep	Overexertion, crashes
Meditation / breathwork	Poor nutrition or alcohol
Red light therapy	Emotional stress
Anti-inflammatory supplements	Sleep deprivation
Gentle movement / stretching	Overtraining

Your **daily HRV score** can show whether your nervous system is **recovering or overwhelmed.**

How to Use HRV With Stimulation

Goal	HRV Strategy
Track taVNS effects	Measure HRV pre- and post-session (optional)
Avoid overdoing it	Skip workouts or stimulation if HRV drops 20%
Test flare triggers	Log HRV drops after activity, diet, stress
Track long-term progress	Weekly or monthly averages rising over time

Think of it like this:

Stimulation trains your vagus nerve—HRV tells you how well it's learning.

Summary: Why HRV Matters

- HRV is a **simple window into your vagal tone and recovery.**

- It improves with **good inputs** like taVNS, breathwork, sleep, and nutrition.

- Watching your HRV helps you **catch problems early** and stay on track.

- It makes recovery **less mysterious** and more measurable.

You don't need to be a data nerd to benefit from HRV. You just need to **start watching your rhythm.**

Your Recovery Dashboard

*How to use HRV, pacing, and vagus stimulation together to heal smarter—
not harder*

You've got the tools:

- HRV tells you how your nervous system is doing.

- PEM tracking tells you how your body handles exertion.

- VNS (and TNS) help retrain your brain–body connection.

But what if you could combine all three—and turn your daily routine into
a real-time feedback system?

In this chapter, you'll learn how to build a **personalized dashboard** that
keeps you **in your recovery zone**, helps you avoid crashes, and shows you
when it's safe to push forward.

Step 1: Track Post-Exertional Malaise (PEM) the Right Way

PEM = delayed crash after activity that was too much for your system. It
can show up hours or even a day later.

What to Track:

Category	Examples
Activity level	Walking, standing, errands, screens, stress
Next-day symptoms	Fatigue, brain fog, HR spikes, flu-like feeling
Recovery time	How many days to return to baseline?

Even a **5-minute journal** or phone note works.

Step 2: Watch HRV Trends—Not Just Daily Numbers

Your **daily HRV** can fluctuate. What matters more:

- Is your **weekly average improving** over time?
- Are there **sharp drops** after certain activities or exposures?
- Does taVNS bring your HRV **up or down**?

When HRV Drops:

- Be cautious. Your system is **overloaded or under-recovered.**
- Reduce stimulation, lower physical/mental load, and sleep more.

When HRV Rises or stabilizes:

- That's your **green light** to gently expand what you're doing.
- Try adding a new therapy (like TNS or red light) or increase gentle movement.

Step 3: Sync Stimulation With Energy Windows

Energy State	What to Do
Feeling OK + HRV stable	Use taVNS in morning + mild movement (walks, yoga)
Low energy but stable HRV	Add breathwork, gentle taVNS, red light
Crashing / low HRV	Rest. Cancel extras. Use left-ear taVNS only.
Stable 5+ days	Add light TNS or second taVNS session carefully

Over time, you'll notice your **"good days" last longer**, and your system tolerates more.

Step 4: Build Your Simple Recovery Dashboard

Create a table like this (daily or weekly):

Day	HRV Score	PEM?	Activity	taVNS Used?	Notes
Mon	32	Yes	Light walk → crash	✔ Morning only	HRV dropped after walk
Tue	24	Yes	Bed rest	✔ Morning	Rested, HRV still low
Wed	31	No	Breathwork + taVNS	✔ Morning + PM	HRV rebounding
Thu	39	No	Red light + walk	✔ Morning	Energy better

This lets you see what's **working**, what's **hurting**, and what's **safe to add**.

Green, Yellow, Red: Use Zones to Stay on Track

Zone	HRV Trend	PEM Symptoms	What to Do
Green	Rising or stable	No crashes	Safely expand: try light exercise or TNS
Yellow	Slight drop	Minor PEM signs	Maintain, don't add more. Increase rest
Red	Drop >15–20%	PEM flare or relapse	Back off, rest, reduce stim time

This system helps prevent **"doing too much on a good day"** which is the classic trap that leads to setback.

Summary: Let the Data Guide You

When you combine:

- **HRV tracking** (internal recovery)

- **PEM monitoring** (external symptom response)

- **VNS/TNS stimulation** (targeted therapy)

...you're no longer flying blind. You're building a **closed feedback loop.** This is like a nervous system GPS that tells you where you are and when it's safe to move.

You're not guessing anymore. You're navigating.

Staying Better for Good

How to keep your progress and what to do if symptoms return

Healing from Long COVID or nervous system dysfunction isn't just about *getting better*—it's about *staying better*. Once you've started to feel more like yourself, this chapter helps you:

- Maintain improvements

- Prevent relapses

- Know what to do if symptoms creep back

- Plan a future that doesn't revolve around fear of crashing

The Recovery Loop: From Survival to Stability

Recovery doesn't happen in a straight line. It's more like a spiral:

1. **Crash**

2. **Stabilize**

3. **Rebuild function**

4. **Expand activity**

5. **Restabilize at a new baseline**

Eventually, you exit the loop. That's the goal of maintenance: keep the gains and avoid sliding back.

Your Maintenance Toolkit

Here's what most people keep in their routine even after major improvement:

Tool	Maintenance Frequency	Why Keep It?
taVNS or TNS	2–4x/week	Keeps vagal tone strong and stable
Breathwork / meditation	Daily or as needed	Supports calm, lowers flare risk
Red light therapy	2–3x/week	Supports mitochondrial and nerve health
Movement (light-moderate)	3–5x/week	Maintains energy capacity + blood flow
Anti-inflammatory diet	80/20 rule	Keeps immune system calm
Sleep routines	Same bedtime + wind-down	Prevents nervous system reactivation

You don't need to do it all forever, just the pieces that keep *you* stable.

What to Do If You Relapse or Flare

Relapses happen. Common triggers include:

- Overexertion
- Infections
- Emotional stress
- Travel, weather shifts, poor sleep

- Skipping support tools for too long

If a flare hits:

1. **Return to daily taVNS**
2. **Add box breathing + limit exertion**
3. **Hydrate + support gut (if GI symptoms return)**
4. **Sleep more, stimulate less (1x/day max)**
5. **Resume tracking until stable again**

Most flares resolve in **3–10 days** if caught early.

Tapering Stimulation Over Time

When you feel 70–90% better, start spacing out your stimulation like this:

Time Since Start	Suggested Frequency
Months 1–2	Daily
Months 3–4	Every other day
Months 5+	2–3x/week or "as needed"

Some people continue taVNS before:

- Flights
- Stressful work weeks
- After colds or vaccinations
- Big social events
- Menstrual cycle phases (for women with hormone sensitivity)

It becomes your **reset button**, not a crutch.

The Full Recovery Mindset

You're not just healing nerves—you're building **resilience**. That means:

- Learning your body's early warning signs
- Knowing how to bring your system back into balance
- Having tools you trust
- Feeling empowered, not fragile

You're not the same person who started this journey. You're more aware, more resourceful, and better equipped to stay well for life.

Final Checklist: Are You Ready to Taper?

I know how to use taVNS and/or TNS correctly

I've seen consistent improvement over at least 4–6 weeks

I'm not relying on stimulation just to survive each day

I've added pacing, breathwork, and diet changes

I have a flare-up plan ready

I feel safe testing less frequent stimulation

If you checked most of these, you're ready to shift from recovery into **maintenance**.

Your New Chapter Begins

You've just completed a full recovery manual—not just for vagus nerve stimulation, but for **nervous system repair**.

Keep these principles close:

- The nervous system is trainable
- Inflammation is reversible
- Healing is not linear

- You are not broken, you're **adaptive**

- Recovery takes time, but *you're in charge now*

Thank you for walking this journey with me. You now have everything you need to continue healing and help others do the same.

Appendix: Getting VNS to Work Without the Frustration

How to set up your vagus nerve stim device, pick the right clip, and fix common problems

If you've gotten this far, you're probably ready to use vagus nerve stimulation (VNS) at home, or maybe you already have. But small things (bad clips, poor contact, wrong settings) can make the difference between results... and nothing.

This appendix gives you exactly what you need to get it working—no guesswork.

Step 1: Choose the Right Device

You do **not** need a $1,000 FDA-cleared device to stimulate your vagus nerve. Many people use a basic **TENS unit** with adjustable frequency and pulse width.

Recommended Budget Device:

- **TENS 7000** or similar with:
  - Adjustable **frequency (Hz)**
  - Adjustable **pulse width (μs)**
  - Can set mode to **"normal" or "continuous"**

Avoid:

- Units that only offer preset "massage" modes
- EMS (Electric Muscle Stimulator) units that twitch muscles—that's not vagal stimulation

Step 2: Pick the Right Ear Clips

You need **2 contact points** to complete the circuit. These can go on:

- The **same ear** (e.g., tragus + concha), or
- **One on the ear**, one on the **neck or shoulder**

Clip Options:

Type	Pros	Cons
Metal ear clips	Strong grip, good conduction	Can pinch or slip, may need wetting
Silicone-coated clips	More comfortable, less pinching	May need **conductive gel** to work
Double clip sets	Easier to set up both contacts on one ear	Not always included with TENS units

Avoid: Alligator clips (too sharp), clips with no rubber pads (can hurt)

Step 3: Target the Right Spot on the Ear

The vagus nerve runs through the **auricular branch**, which reaches:

- **Tragus** (small flap near ear canal)
- **Cymba concha** (upper inner bowl of ear)
- **Cavum concha** (lower inner bowl of ear)

Best Starting Point:

- **Left tragus**: easiest to clip, minimal heart risk
- Avoid: **Earlobe** as it's not innervated by the vagus nerve

Step 4: Program the Settings

Setting	What to Use (for taVNS)
Mode	"Normal" or "Continuous"
Frequency (Hz)	25 Hz (range: 15–30 Hz is acceptable)
Pulse Width	250 microseconds (µs)
Intensity	Mild tingle or warmth (no pain or twitching)
Session Time	15–30 minutes
Side	Start with **left ear** only

Use once daily at first. If well tolerated, increase to **2x/day**.

Troubleshooting Guide

Problem	Fix
No sensation	Wet the ear slightly or use saline gel
Painful or sharp feeling	Lower intensity and/or switch to soft clip
No heart rate response	Check placement and/or increase session length
Tingling stops mid-session	Adjust clips or re-wet area
Symptoms worsen after session	Use shorter time and/or lower intensity
Lightheadedness / bradycardia (slow heart rate)	Avoid right ear, especially in POTS patients

Conductive Gel Tips

You don't need fancy gel. Try:

- Saline eye drops
- Contact lens solution
- Store-bought TENS conductive gel (e.g., Spectra)

Apply a small drop to each clip point before placing the electrode.

Sample Weekly Plan (First Month)

Week	Frequency	Session Time	Intensity Level
1	1x/day	15 min	Low
2	1x/day	20–30 min	Low-moderate
3	2x/day	20–30 min	Moderate
4	Adjust as needed	Based on results	Comfortable tingling only

Monitor symptoms, energy, HRV, and PEM risk weekly.

Final Tips

- **No muscle twitching** = correct stimulation

- **Use same time daily** for consistency

- **Don't stimulate during a crash** or fever

- If you feel worse after multiple tries, **pause** and reassess placement or settings

References

Acanfora D, Nolano M, Acanfora C, Colella C, Provitera V, Caporaso G, Rodolico GR, Bortone AS, Galasso G, Casucci G. Impaired Vagal Activity in Long-COVID-19 Patients. Viruses. 2022 May 13;14(5):1035. DOI: 10.3390/v14051035. PMID: 35632776; PMCID: PMC9147759.

Badran, B. W., Huffman, S. M., Dancy, M., Austelle, C. W., & 3 more. (n.d.). A pilot randomized controlled trial of supervised, at-home, self-administered transcutaneous auricular vagus nerve stimulation (taVNS) to manage Long COVID symptoms. *Preprint.*

Bonaz, B., Sinniger, V., Pellissier, S., Clarençon, D., Mathieu, N., & Dantzer, C. (2016). Vagus nerve stimulation: A new promising therapeutic tool in inflammatory bowel disease. Journal of Internal Medicine, 280(1), 51–63.

Bremner, J. D., Gurel, N. Z., Wittbrodt, M. T., Shandhi, M. M. H., Rapaport, M. H., & Kilpatrick, D. G. (2020).

Bretherton, B., Atkinson, L., Murray, A., Clancy, J., Deuchars, S. A., & Deuchars, J. (2019). Effects of transcutaneous vagus nerve stimulation in individuals aged 55 years or above: Potential benefits of daily stimulation. Aging, 11(14), 4836–4857. Transcutaneous cervical vagal nerve stimulation reduces sympathetic nerve activity in posttraumatic stress disorder: A randomized, double-blind, sham-controlled trial. Neurobiology of Stress, 13, 100254.

Dani M, Dirksen A, Taraborrelli P, Torocastro M, Panagopoulos D, Sutton R, Lim PB. Autonomic dysfunction in 'Long COVID': rationale, physiology and management strategies. Clin Med (Lond). 2021 Jan;21(1):e63-e67. DOI: 10.7861/clinmed.2020-0896. Epub 2020 Nov 26.

Dawson, J., Pierce, D., Dixit, A., Kimberley, T. J., Robertson, M., Tarver, B., ... & Engineer, N. D. (2021). Vagus nerve stimulation paired with rehabilitation for upper limb motor function after ischemic stroke (VNS-REHAB): A randomized, blinded, pivotal, device trial. The Lancet, 397(10284), 1545–1553.

Englot, D. J., Chang, E. F., & Auguste, K. I. (2011). Vagus nerve stimulation for epilepsy: A meta-analysis of efficacy and predictors of response. Journal of Neurosurgery, 115(6), 1248–1255.

García de Gurtubay, I., Bermejo, P., López, M., Larraya, I., & Librero, J. (2021). Evaluation of different vagus nerve stimulation anatomical targets in the ear by vagus evoked potential responses. Brain and Behavior, 11(11), e2343.

George, M. S., Ward, H. E., Ninan, P. T., Pollack, M., Nahas, Z., Anderson, B., ... & Ballenger, J. C. (2008). A pilot study of vagus nerve stimulation (VNS) for treatment-resistant anxiety disorders. Brain Stimulation, 1(2), 112–121.

Goadsby, P. J., Grosberg, B. M., Mauskop, A., Cady, R. K., Simmons, K. A., & Saper, J. R. (2018). Non-invasive vagus nerve stimulation for the acute treatment of episodic and chronic cluster headache: A randomized, double-blind, sham-controlled ACT2 study. Cephalalgia, 38(5), 959–969.

González-Rosa, J. J., & García-Muñoz, C. (2021). Noninvasive vagus nerve stimulation in Parkinson's disease: Current perspectives. Expert Review of Neurotherapeutics, 21(10), 1111–1121.

Gurel, N. Z., Wittbrodt, M. T., & Bremner, J. D. (2022). Effects of noninvasive cervical vagal nerve stimulation on executive function in healthy adults: A randomized, sham-controlled study. Brain Stimulation, 15(4), 1020–1027.

He, W., Wang, X., Shi, H., Shang, H., & Wang, X. (2012). Auricular acupuncture and its effect on autonomic nervous regulation: A review. Autonomic Neuroscience: Basic and Clinical, 157(1–2), 63–68.

Jigo, M., Carmel, J. B., Wang, Q., & Rodenkirch, C. (2024). Transcutaneous cervical vagus nerve stimulation improves sensory performance in humans: A randomized controlled crossover pilot study. Scientific Reports, 14(1), 3975.

Khan, M. W. Z., Ahmad, M., Qudrat, S., Afridi, F., & Khan, N. A. (2024). Vagal nerve stimulation for the management of long COVID symptoms. Infectious Medicine, 3(4), 234–238.

Lehrer, P. M., et al. (2020). Heart rate variability biofeedback improves health outcomes. Frontiers in Psychology, 11, 571691.

Liu, A., Song, L., Li, L., Wang, X., & Lin, H. (2014). A controlled trial of transcutaneous vagus nerve stimulation for the treatment of pharmacoresistant epilepsy. Epilepsy & Behavior, 39, 105–110.

Möller, M., Schroeder, C. F., & May, A. (2018). Vagus nerve stimulation modulates the cranial trigeminal autonomic reflex. Annals of Neurology, 84(6), 886–892.

Natelson, B. H., Blate, M., & Soto, T. (2023). Transcutaneous vagus nerve stimulation in the treatment of Long COVID-chronic fatigue syndrome. Archives of Clinical and Biomedical Research, 7(2), 89-98.

Özden, A. V., & Perçin, A. (n.d.). A promising method for post-COVID/Long-COVID syndrome: Noninvasive vagus nerve stimulation. *Bahçeşehir University* and *Iğdır University*.

Powell, K., Lin, K., Tambo, W. et al. Trigeminal nerve stimulation: a current state-of-the-art review. Bioelectron Med 9, 30 (2023).

Rush, A. J., George, M. S., Sackeim, H. A., Marangell, L. B., Husain, M. M., Giller, C., ... & Nahas, Z. (2000). Vagus nerve stimulation (VNS) for treatment-resistant depressions: A multicenter study. Biological Psychiatry, 47(4), 276–286.

Sigrist, C., Torki, B., Bolz, L.-O., Jeglorz, T., & Bolz, A. (2023). Transcutaneous auricular vagus nerve stimulation in pediatric patients: A systematic review of clinical treatment protocols and stimulation parameters. Neuromodulation: Technology at the Neural Interface, 26(3), 345–356.

Stavrakis, S., Humphrey, M. B., Scherlag, B. J., Hu, Y., Jackman, W. M., Nakagawa, H., & Lazzara, R. (2015). Low-level transcutaneous electrical vagus nerve stimulation suppresses atrial fibrillation. Journal of the American College of Cardiology, 65(9), 867–875.

Straube, A., Ellrich, J., Eren, O., Blum, B., & Ruscheweyh, R. (2015). Treatment of chronic migraine with transcutaneous stimulation of the auricular branch of the vagal nerve (auricular t-VNS): A randomized, monocentric clinical trial. The Journal of Headache and Pain, 16, 543.

Tavares-Figueiredo, I., Pers, Y.-M., Duflos, C., Herman, F., Sztajnzalc, B., Lecoq, H., Laffont, I., Dupeyron, A. F., & Homs, A. F. (2024). Effect of transcutaneous auricular vagus nerve stimulation in chronic low back pain: A pilot study. Journal of Clinical Medicine, 13(24), 7601.

Torres-Rosas, R., Yehia, G., Peña, G., Mishra, P., del Rocio Thompson-Bonilla, M., Moreno-Eutimio, M. A., ... & Ulloa, L. (2014).

Dopamine mediates vagal modulation of the immune system by electroacupuncture. Nature Medicine, 20(3), 291–295.

Tracey, K. J., & Pavlov, V. A. (2017). A neural basis for the inflammatory reflex. Nature Reviews Immunology, 17(6), 391–404.

Verbanck, P., Clarinval, A. M., Burton, F., Corazza, F., Nagant, C., & Cheron, G. (2021). Transcutaneous auricular vagus nerve stimulation (tVNS) can reverse the manifestations of the Long-COVID syndrome: A pilot study. *Journal of Neurophysiology & Movement Biomechanics, Université Libre de Bruxelles.*

Wang, H., Shi, S., Guo, T., & Zhang, Y. (2015). Effects of acupuncture on vagal regulation of gastrointestinal motility. Journal of Gastrointestinal Disorders, 21(3), 192–199.

Wang, M.-X., Wumiti, A., Gao, X.-S., Zhang, Y.-M., Zhang, Z.-P., Peng, Y.-M., & Zhang, H.-M. (2023). Transcutaneous cervical vagus nerve stimulation improved motor cortex excitability in healthy adults: A randomized, single-blind, self-crossover design study. Frontiers in Neuroscience, 17, 1234033.

Wu, Y., Song, L., Wang, X., Li, N., Zhan, S., Rong, P., Wang, Y., & Liu, A. (2022). Transcutaneous vagus nerve stimulation could improve the effective rate on the quality of sleep in the treatment of primary insomnia: A randomized control trial. Brain Sciences, 12(10), 1296.

Yap, J. Y. Y., Keatch, C., Lambert, E., Woods, W., Stoddart, P. R., & Kameneva, T. (2020). Critical review of transcutaneous vagus nerve stimulation: Challenges for translation to clinical practice. Frontiers in Neuroscience, 14, Article 284.

Yuan, H., & Silberstein, S. D. (2016). Vagus nerve and vagus nerve stimulation, a comprehensive review: Part II. Headache: The Journal of Head and Face Pain, 56(2), 259-266.

Zhang, S., Zhao, Y., Qin, Z., Han, Y., He, J., Zhao, B., Wang, L., Duan, Y., Huo, J., Wang, T., & Wang, Y. (2024). Transcutaneous auricular vagus nerve stimulation for chronic insomnia disorder: A randomized clinical trial. JAMA Network Open, 7(12), e2451217.

Zhao, B., Wang, P., Dong, C., et al. (2012). Auricular acupuncture reduces systemic inflammation via vagus nerve activation. Brain, Behavior, and Immunity, 26(1), 23–31.

www.ingramcontent.com/pod-product-compliance
Lightning Source LLC
Chambersburg PA
CBHW060227030426
42335CB00014B/1362